ALOE VERA

The Natural Healing Choice

ALOE VERA

The Natural Healing Choice

Lee Faber

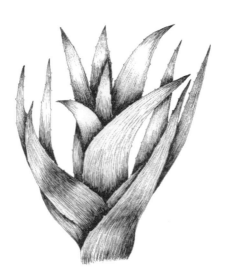

Abbeydale Press

ISBN 978-1-86147-237-3

1 3 5 7 9 10 8 6 4 2

Published by Abbeydale Press
an imprint of Bookmart Ltd
Registered number 2372865
Trading as Bookmart Ltd
Blaby Road, Wigston, Leicester
LE18 4SE, England

Produced by Omnipress Limited, UK
Illustrations by Tegan Sharrard
Cover design by Omnipress Limited

Printed in Dubai

ABOUT THE AUTHOR

Lee Faber is an American who became a British citizen, having
been in the UK since 1981. She has lived and worked in New
York, Florida, London and now resides in Wiltshire.

During her career she has been involved in book editing and
writing with an emphasis on health, food and cookery. She has
specialised in Americanising/Anglicising books on a variety of
subjects for both US and UK publishers.

She is an accomplished cook and has created many recipes.

Lee has written another book in this series, *Healthy Oils*.

CONTENTS

Disclaimer

There are numerous claims made as to the benefits of Aloe Vera and while there is a lot of ongoing clinical research currently being undertaken, there are probably as many disclaimers as there are claims. The majority of individuals and organisations seem to agree, however, that Aloe Vera is effective as a laxative and for its skin soothing properties. No one has yet proved its efficacy in the treatment of disease.

Introduction

As you will discover from reading this book, Aloe Vera is used for an enormous number of beneficial, health-giving and curative applications. It is indeed a 'Pharmacy in a Plant'.

Despite the fact that only a few of its uses have been scientifically authenticated, unlike some medicinal herbs and plants, the global cultivation of the Aloe Vera plant is enormous.

Worldwide, over 50,000 acres are used to cultivate Aloe Vera, with Central American countries being by far the largest producers. These countries are capable of increasing their growing areas manyfold, so there is no likelihood of usage outpacing cultivation.

Global sales of Aloe Vera and products containing it amount to millions of pounds sterling, and the uses are expanding all the time.

It might surprise you to learn that you can grow Aloe Vera in your own home and enjoy many of its benefits from the plant itself.

The virtues of Aloe have been written about for centuries. One of the foremost figures in herbal medicine was Nicholas Culpeper (1616–1654). His works, although dismissed by certain medical historians, came to prominence in the latter half of the 20th century as people looked for alternative cures for their ailments that could not be found in advancements in science. Culpeper's *Complete Herbal*, published in 1653, had this to say about Aloe (it was not the same variety of Aloe as the one we discuss in this book, but his description is very much the same as that used today):

ALOES
Names. *Called also sea houseleek, and sea-ay-green.*

Description. *This plant has very long leaves, thick and set round about with short points or crests, standing* wide one from another: the root is thick and long; all the herb is of a strong flavour and bitter taste. Out of this herb is drawn a juice which is dried and called Aloes, after the plant Aloe, in different parts of the world. There are three sorts of Aloes common in the shops, but that which is procured from this plant, and distinguished by the name of Succotrine Aloes, is by far the best for internal use.

Place. It grows very plentifully in India, and the best juice is brought from thence: it also grows in many places of Asia and Arabia, near the sea side.

Government and virtues. It is a martial plant, hot in the second degree, and dry in the third; of a very bitter taste; the juice being refined and clarified from its dross, is of a clear and blackish clean brown colour: it opens the belly, and purges cold, phlegmatic, and choleric humours which overburden and hurt the stomach: it is the basis in almost all pills and comforts, cleanses and dries up all superfluous humours. It may be taken with cinnamon, ginger, mace, galangal, or aniseed, to assuage and drive away pains of the stomach, to warm it and expel phlegm: the same is also good against the jaundice and spitting of blood. Aloes made into powder, and strewed upon new bloody wounds, stops the blood and heals them: it likewise closes up old ulcers, particularly those about the private parts and fundament: boiled with wine and honey, it heals rifts and haemorrhoids: applied with honey it takes away black spots that come by stripes or bruises, and is good against inflammations, hurts, and scabs of the eyes, and against running and dimness of the same. Mixed with oil of roses and vinegar, and applied to the forehead and temples, it helps the head-ache: the head being rubbed with Aloes mixed with wine, preserves the hair; applied with wine, it cures sore mouths, sore gums, sore throat, and kernels under the tongue, and outwardly applied, is a good consolidative medicine. It likewise powerfully resists putrefaction, removes obstructions of the viscera, kills worms in the stomach and intestines, is good for the ague, green sickness, and provokes the menses.

What is
Aloe Vera?

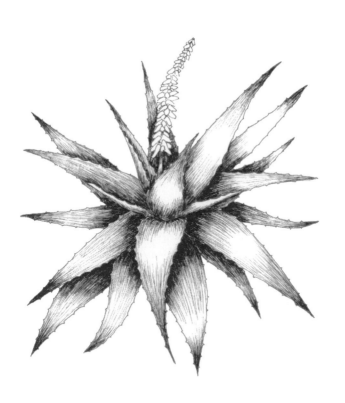

The Aloe Vera plant, *Aloe barbadensis*, is a cactus-like perennial in the lily family known for its healing and soothing properties. The thick, succulent leaves are pale greyish-green with lighter spots and points along the edges. The centre of each leaf is filled with a viscous gel. While Aloe Vera seldom blooms as a houseplant, when grown outdoors or in a warm greenhouse, it will produce tall stalks of 1 inch-long green, white, yellow or orange flowers. Aloe Vera is often referred to as the 'first aid' plant because of its ability to soothe irritated skin, especially sunburned skin. (Other references to Aloe Vera call it a 'medicine plant' or a 'burn plant'.)

Aloe Vera is also a gentle, soothing anti-inflammatory, antimicrobial and antifungal ingredient used in a long list of cosmetics: shampoos, moisturisers, aftershaves, lipsticks, lotions and creams, household cleansers, babies' nappies, women's tights, latex examination gloves and other products.

FORMS OF ALOE VERA

FROM THE GROWING PLANT
Diagram of a sliced Aloe Vera leaf showing the outer skin, gel and latex sections.

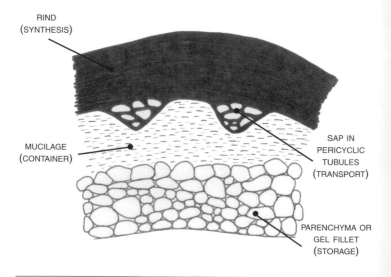

Aloe Vera is a complex plant made up of many constituent parts including vitamins, amino acids, enzymes and mono- and polysaccharides. These are what give Aloe Vera its many healing properties. The rind is the manufacturing plant for carbohydrates, fats, proteins and vitamins. Below the rind are vascular bundles of xylem and phloem. This is the sap, or transport system of the plant, which takes up water and minerals from the roots and transports the products of photosynthesis to be stored in the gel. Mucilage was once thought to take part in this transport process, but researchers now feel that it acts as a container for the gel fillet or the storage of Aloe Vera. The plant is usually separated into two products: gel and latex.

ALOE VERA GEL
This is found in the inner leaf of the growing plant: the parenchyma tissues. It is a known anti-inflammatory and also has antibacterial and antifungal properties. It is most commonly used for minor cuts and burns as a healer and pain reliever.

ALOE VERA LATEX
The latex, sometimes referred to as the 'sap' or 'juice', is a bitter, yellow sticky substance from the pericyclic tubules found just beneath the outer skin of the leaf surface. It is well-known in pharmaceutical use as a laxative which is, to date, the only fully authenticated use. But, a word of warning . . . this liquid is potent! Don't let it get mixed in with your transparent gel. And don't consider ingesting the sap if you are menstruating, pregnant, breastfeeding, have kidney disease or have a tendency to get haemorrhoids. (The potion also tastes incredibly bitter. In fact, some Jamaican mothers will dab a bit on their breasts when they want to instantly wean their children.)

My sister, who now lives in the Caribbean, says Aloe Vera plants are grown by people all over the islands and used for everything that ails you — being dabbed on, eaten, drunk and chewed. It is her view that the natives who are 'used to' the plant, react less violently to the effects of the latex than those who are new converts.

RETAIL PRODUCTS

The most fitting description about what type of Aloe to use, according to the American physician Dr Ivan Danhof, is: 'The best aloe is a preparation which maximises the desired constituents, minimises any ingredient with negative effects, maintains the constituents in an unaltered and active form, preserves the actions and benefits and is present in the final product in amounts which, indeed, can bring about the desired result when the product is used as recommended.'

For internal use, the best form of aloe is 100% pure stabilised Aloe Vera gel taken as a health drink. This stabilised gel should also be the major ingredient of any product applied to the skin. If a product is clear, looks like water and tastes like water, it probably is water and will not be particularly beneficial.

To produce Aloe Vera gel, the mature leaves of Aloe Vera are harvested when the plant is about four years old. The product is produced either from the whole leaf, which is ground up and filtered to remove the solid matter, passing through carbon filters to extract all the anthraquinone (a yellow crystalline powder that is insoluble in water and used chiefly in the manufacture of dyes), or the parenchymal plant tissue, and the mucilage is filleted out of the leaf to produce a gel containing only a tiny amount of sap.

The product is then preserved or 'stabilised' by subjecting it to either heat or chemical sterilisation. Various antioxidants are often added which protect the product. Preservatives, thickening and flavouring agents also help stabilise the end product by preventing contamination and chemical and physical change.
In commercial products, the terms 'gel', 'juice', 'sap' and 'latex' are not always clearly defined by manufacturers and are often confused by consumers. Mechanical separation is not always perfect, so Aloe latex is sometimes found in some Aloe gels. It is desirable to make the gel as pure as possible, because Aloe latex contains the anthraquinone glycosides aloin A and B which are potent laxatives.

ALOE VERA CREAMS AND LOTIONS are available to protect and moisturise dry and irritated skin.

ALOE VERA GEL in a tube helps soothe irritations caused by overexposure to the sun.

ALOE VERA JUICE, produced from the gel, is often helpful in cases of digestive disorders and for detoxification programmes. It doesn't taste very nice, so many retailers are mixing 100% pure Aloe Vera gel with fruit flavours such as cranberry to make it more palatable.

Which brings up something else. There really isn't any 100% pure Aloe Vera sold. If 100% pure Aloe Vera juice was to go out for distribution it would rot or ferment long before reaching the point of sale. This means that any liquid product on the market that claims to be '100% Aloe Vera' cannot be genuinely quite 100%, although it can be very nearly so. And any liquid product that claims to have 'no preservatives' has got to be wrong unless it were tinned or otherwise sterilised or was on very short-term distribution — rather like fresh milk. Hence the preservatives are unavoidable.

There is also the practice of describing a product as being 'made with 100% Aloe Vera'. This will usually mean that some percentage of the total product will be composed of 100% Aloe Vera, but there will be other ingredients as well and the Aloe Vera component may be quite small. This could, and does, easily mislead the uninitiated. So, some preservatives are needed even if the Aloe extract is genuinely from the plant and hasn't been contaminated with anything else, otherwise the extract couldn't possibly be stabilised for distribution and marketing. The consumer wants to see the amount of preservatives kept to a minimum and be sure that only the most benign preservatives are used. The most important thing is that full disclosure should be given so that it is clear to the consumer what he or she is buying.

ALOE VERA TABLETS AND CAPSULES The benefits of Aloe Vera can be received as capsules, too. These capsules contain Aloe Vera juice in a freeze-dried form. As a food supplement, Aloe Vera capsules are said to aid blood and lymphatic circulation and facilitate digestion. They are sold in health food shops in a variety of dosages for people who do not care for the taste of the juice or want a more convenient means of taking Aloe Vera.

Commercial products containing Aloe Vera include shampoos and conditioners, shaving cream, aftershave, lip creams, sunscreens, toothpastes, slimming aids, food supplements, antifungal treatments, depilators and examination gloves, with more products being added all the time.

I'm a recent convert to Aloe Vera. Years ago I was visiting some friends in Florida and got sunburnt. One friend broke a leaf off an Aloe plant growing in her garden and suggested that I try putting the gel on the worst bits. Unfortunately, I reacted badly to it and broke out in a rash which put me off the whole idea. But I kept hearing such good things about Aloe Vera that it occurred to me it might not have been the right sort of Aloe or I might have been applying latex rather than gel. I thought I ought to give it another try. I haven't had sunburn recently, but Aloe Vera shampoo and conditioner (the brand I tried also contains jojoba) make my hair noticeably brighter in colour, glossy and healthy looking. And the tooth gel containing natural peppermint and spearmint flavours makes my mouth feel extra clean and fresh. I have also tried the multipurpose gel in a tube on small wounds, because my plants aren't mature enough yet to use, and have been very satisfied with the results.

When buying Aloe Vera products it is important to use those that are as pure and natural as possible. So be sure to read product labels and understand what you might be putting onto or into your body.

There are several suppliers of certified organic Aloe Vera, but to the best of my knowledge, the Carrington lab subsidiary in Costa Rica is the only Aloe Vera farming operation that is certified by Eco-Logica (an accredited certifying body recognised by the USDA, the EU and the government of Switzerland) as being organic and

manufactured in a kosher and ISO-certified facility that is current good manufacturing practice (cGMP) by the FDA and, for an injectable biologic, by the USDA. According to the International Aloe Science Council (IASC), only some members are certified, but not all members provide documentation supporting their organic certification.
The International Aloe Science Council is an independent organisation in the USA that evaluates the quality of Aloe products. If the products meet certain criteria and reach the minimum standard set by the council, they are accredited with the IASC seal of approval. This seal can then be displayed on the product. It makes sense to buy products that contain this seal. As of July 2007, 95 companies that grow, process, manufacture or market Aloe Vera throughout the world are certified. You can check them out by going to:

http://www.iasc.org/complete.html#B

Growing
Aloe Vera

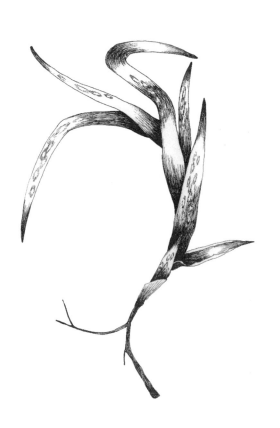

I have always thought of Aloe Vera as a tropical plant, but it can be purchased from nurseries and garden centres in the UK and grown successfully here. Or, if you have a friend who has an Aloe Vera plant, you might be able to coax them in to giving you a cutting. Propagate from small, rooted offshoots at the base of the parent plant when they are a couple of inches tall (or larger).

There is an added bonus to Aloe Vera — you can grow it indoors. No green fingers are required. I'm certainly not a gardener, but I have three Aloe plants growing on my windowsills in varying stages of growth and they are all very healthy. I have even repotted one without killing it off. Aloe Vera is attractive and easy to maintain and when you want to try some of its magic, just break off a piece! Rub the gel on your skin or throw some into fruit juice. It is also easy to add Aloe Vera gel to homemade smoothies or freshly squeezed juices. If you are using it internally, according to the experts you should wait until the plant is mature — three to four years old — by which time its leaves will be about 60 centimetres (about 24 inches) in length and about 8 centimetres (3 inches) wide at the base of the leaf.

Aloes like a south-facing position: a front porch, near a sunny window or similar, but will tolerate partial shade. Choose a pot with a drainage hole or provide a 2.5—5 centimetres (1—2 inch) layer of gravel in the bottom of the pot. Plant in sandy compost: commercial potting compost with extra perlite, granite, grit or coarse sand added. Alternatively, use a potting mix specifically for cactus plants. The Aloe Vera should soon multiply and

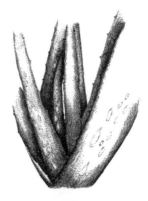

grow flowers after a couple of years. As the plant grows, the pot should also grow progressively larger. It is best to leave your Aloe plant in the pot and place it near a window that gets a lot of sun.

Fertilise annually in the spring with a half-strength bloom-type fertiliser with NPK 10–40–10. You can move the pot outdoors during the summer months. Aloe Vera is a succulent and as such, stores a large quantity of water within its leaves and root system. During the summer the soil should be completely soaked, but then allowed to dry out again before re-watering.
Aloes have a shallow, spreading root system, so when it is time to repot, choose a wide planter rather than a deep one. Little baby Aloes will pop up near the base of the plant. When grown indoors the offshoots can be removed and repotted when they are a few inches tall.

Aloe Vera cannot tolerate either severe heat or cold (lower than 5°C/40°F). In the winter the plant will become somewhat dormant and will utilise little moisture, so during this period watering should be minimal. Allow the soil to become completely dry before adding water.

HOW TO REVIVE AN AILING PLANT
If you are overwatering your Aloe Vera plant or if it looks like it is ailing, here is how to revive it.

Place the plant in the corner of a sunny room as close to the light as possible. Allow the soil to dry out between waterings. Remember that Aloe is a succulent, similar to cactus.

Or, plant the Aloe Vera in a clay pot and wedge the plant into a slightly larger nonporous pot that you have filled with a little water, ensuring that there is air space between the water and your plant pot and that there is always a little water in the larger pot. The water provides sufficient humidity for the Aloe's needs without risking root rot. This method also produces good results for establishing new plants from offshoots with no roots.

Fertilise with a half-strength liquid fertiliser solution, prepared using packet directions. The Aloe Vera may have exhausted its nutrient supply if it has been in the same container for more than a few years.

Aloe Vera has a lifespan of about 12 years, although the leaves are usually harvested when the plant is three to four years old. When the outer leaves are severed, the plant is able to seal itself. The cut covers itself very quickly, first with a thin film, and then with a rubbery protective coating which prevents the stem from drying out and enables the plant to continue living. Soon the 'wound' heals completely. No wonder it has been called 'the medicine plant'.

History of
Aloe Vera

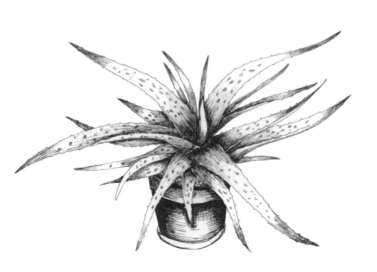

Imagine you lived 4,000 years ago. You are very hungry. You come across a spiny plant sticking out of the ground that you've never seen before and you think to yourself, 'Hmmm, this looks delicious. I wonder what it tastes like.' You break off a piece and taste it. It's very bitter, and not at all delicious so you spit it out. Then you notice you've got some jelly stuff stuck on your hands. Do you think, 'If I rub some of this gooey stuff on my skin, I wonder whether it'll make my sunburnt skin feel better?'

How DID people discover what was safe to eat and what other properties the plant might have? Trial and error? If you tasted something and you didn't get ill or die, did you assume it was all right? And how was it determined which plants were good for your skin? Was it all accidental?

It took early man thousands of years to develop an understanding of plants, of what can and cannot be consumed, of what will heal and what will harm. Many of our over-the-counter medicines are distillations, combinations, reproductions or variations of substances found in nature. Some of these substances were recommended by our forefathers long before their value was demonstrated and understood through scientific research.

Aloe Vera has a venerable history. For over 3,500 years, tales of healing Aloe Vera plants have been handed down through centuries by word of mouth. From the Bible's mention of removing Christ from the Cross and wrapping his body in aloes and myrrh (John 19:39, 19:40 *'And there came also Nicodemus, which at the first came to Jesus by night, and brought a mixture of myrrh and aloes, about an hundred pound weight. Then took they the body of Jesus, and wound it in linen clothes with the spices, as the manner of the Jews is to bury.'*), we find Aloe Vera mysteriously appearing in every phase of history, with many testimonials to its great medicinal value. It is now thought that this wasn't really Aloe Vera that was mentioned in the Bible, but another form of Aloe, prized for making incense and embalming fluid.

The earliest documented use of Aloe Vera comes from the ancient Egyptians, but it was also grown and used by King Solomon, who was said to have valued it highly.

Most botanists agree, backed by historical evidence, that the Aloe Vera plant originated in the warm, dry climate of northern Africa. However, because the plant is so adaptable, and because man has been so eager to carry it with him from place to place, it can now be found in many warm countries.

One myth (or it may be a fact) is that Alexander the Great, after conquering Persia in 333 BC, was said to have been persuaded by his mentor Aristotle, to capture the island of Socotra in the Indian Ocean. This battle was fought in order to secure the island's famed Aloe supplies that were needed to treat Alexander's wounded soldiers.

One of the earliest books on the subject of natural medicine (the only kind of medicine around at the time) was the *Rig Veda*, compiled in India sometime between 1700 and 1100 BC (the early Vedic period), which lists hundreds of plants deemed useful in the treatment of diseases.

In Sumer, a very early civilisation in Mesopotamia, later called Babylonia, archaeologists have located in the city of Nippur the site of the Qula temple, one of the oldest temples for medication and treatment of diseases. Excavations at this site have yielded thousands of clay tablets with contents that show botanical sources for animal and plant substances used for healing.

The first detailed discussion of Aloe Vera's medicinal value is probably that which is found in an Egyptian document written around 1550 BC. This document gives 12 formulas for mixing Aloe Vera with other agents to treat both internal and external human disorders.

A milestone in Western man's detailed understanding of medicinal plants is the work of Hippocrates (460–375 BC), the father of modern medicine. (Doctors today still take the Hippocratic Oath.) His *Materia Medica* makes no direct mention of Aloe Vera, but during that same period, the plant, according to Copra's *Indigenous Drugs of India*, had come into widespread use. Interestingly, Copra writes, 'The use of Aloes, the common musabbar (if dried in the sun, the Aloe Vera gel turns into a wax-like non-transparent blackish substance called kumarisar or musabbar), for external application to inflamed painful parts of the body and for causing purgation (internal cleansing) is too well known in India to need any special mention.'

Materia Medica is a Latin term for the body of collected knowledge about the therapeutic properties of any substance used for healing; what we would call a drug. The term was used from the period of the Roman Empire until the 20th century, but has now been generally replaced in medical education contexts with the word pharmacology, except within homeopathy, where it remains current. In Latin, the term literally means 'medical matters'.

One of the most well-known early uses of the term was as the title of a work by the Greek pharmaco-botanist Dioscorides in the first century AD, *Materia Medica Libri Quinque* (concerning medical matters in five volumes). This famous commentary covered about 600 plant drugs plus a number of therapeutically useful animal and mineral products. Dioscorides developed his knowledge and skill as he travelled with that great empire's armies. He gave the first detailed description of Aloe Vera, and attributed to its juices 'the power of binding, of inducing sleep'. He noted as well that it 'loosens the belly, cleansing the stomach'. He further added that this 'bitter' Aloe (the sap) was a treatment for boils; that it eased haemorrhoids; that it aided in healing bruises; that it was good for the tonsils, the gums, and all general mouth irritations; and that it worked as a medicine for the eyes. Dioscorides further observed that the whole leaf, when pulverised, could stop the bleeding of many wounds.

Materia Medica Libri Quinque is a precursor to all modern pharmacopeias and is one of the most influential herbal books in history. In fact it remained in use until about AD 1600. Unlike many other classical authors, Dioscorides' work was not 'rediscovered' in the Renaissance because his book never left circulation. The *Materia Medica* was often reproduced in manuscript form through the centuries, often with commentary on Dioscorides' work and with minor additions.

In Greek pharmacology, the plant was first mentioned by Celsius (25 BC—AD 50), but his comments were limited to its power as a purgative.

The earliest description of the manufacture of drug Aloes comes from the 9th-century Persian merchant Abu Hanifeh, who reported the production of Arabian Aloes from *Aloe barbadensis*. The Arabs crushed and threw mature leaves into presses, where they were trodden until the juice flowed. The mass was then left to thicken, put into leather bags and exposed to the sun until dry. Later manufacturing methods are not a great deal more sophisticated.

During his fabled travels in the Orient, among the many marvels recorded by Marco Polo (1254—1324), probably the most famous Western traveller on the Silk Road in the Orient, were his descriptions of the many applications of the Aloe Vera plant. And Christopher Columbus in his travels also documented the use of Aloe Vera as an important medicine.

The virtues of Aloe Vera have been recorded by many great civilisations, from Persia and Egypt in the Middle East, to Greece and Italy in Europe, and India and the African continent. The plant is widely known in Asia and the Pacific and is found in the folklore of the Japanese, the Philippines and the Hawaiians. The Spanish used Aloe and carried it with them to their new world colonies in South America and the Caribbean islands.

The Spanish Conquistadors discovered various herbal medicines in use in Tenochtitlán, the Aztecs' capital city. It is known that Aloe Vera was the effective agent at the heart of many of the Aztec cures, it is known that Aloe Vera was the effective agent. During the 16th century, the Spanish transported these Aztec herbal medecines back to Europe, where they became the foundation for modern Western medicine.

Aloe Vera was brought to the New World by Spanish missionaries. It was planted around Catholic missions and used extensively by the missionaries and the native population as a universal healing agent throughout the Caribbean islands, Central and South America. It was developed as a commercial crop by the Spanish, particularly on the island of Barbados, and by the Dutch, mainly on the island of Curacao. The sap was extracted from the plant and boiled down into a black mass for export, mainly to Europe.

The Swedish Scientist Carl Linnaeus, also known as Carl von Linné or Carolus Linnaeus, is often called the Father of Taxonomy. His system for naming, ranking and classifying organisms is still in wide use today, albeit with many changes. His ideas on classification have influenced generations of biologists during and after his lifetime, even those opposed to the philosophical and theological roots of his work. In 1720, he was the first to name *Aloe Vera Linne*, the plant we call Aloe Vera, which is also referred to today as *Aloe Barbadensis Miller*.

Aloe Vera found its way to England in the late 17th century and remained a very popular prescribed and over-the-counter medicine throughout the 18th and 19th centuries, but it took until the 1850s for T. & H. Smith in Edinburgh to discover aloin in the latex component of Aloe Vera, which they determined was a digestive tonic in small doses and a very powerful laxative in larger doses. Aside from being used as a laxative, Aloe latex was also used to expel intestinal worms.

Over the centuries hundreds of papers and references have been published by physicians and laymen worldwide describing Aloe Vera's many uses as a healing agent. Aloe Vera was officially listed as a purgative and a skin protectant by the United States Pharmacopoeia (USP) in 1820.

In the 20th century, the first commercial US Aloe Vera farm was established in Florida in 1912.

Modern use of Aloe Vera was first documented in the 1930s to heal radiation burns: a paper by C. E. Collins described the use of the whole Aloe leaf to heal radiation dermatitis on the forehead of a 31-year-old female, stating that the skin returned to normal with little or no scarring and normal skin colour. Collins and son did a study on 50 patients with radiation injuries, burns, ulcers and dermatitis, in which all were successfully healed. They used Aloe Vera leaf split in half or an ointment made from a combination of the sap and gel. The ointment was described as having a yellow colour and an offensive odour.

It was also used after the Second World War to aid the victims of the fallout in Nagasaki and Hiroshima. It was reported that the victims who were treated with Aloe Vera showed signs of increased tissue growth and reduced pain, where other medicines had failed.

In 1945 there was a Russian report stating that boiled Aloe juice was a very effective treatment for a skin disease caused by parasites. It also adds that drinking Aloe juice is an effective treatment for many types of lung disorders.

The work continued all over the world, with claims being made that Aloe Vera was effective in curing skin injuries faster than any other treatment; that the boiled sap killed tuberculosis bacteria and treated ulcers, radiation and fire burns, frostbite, cuts and blisters; that it greatly improved skin texture, and eliminated dryness, itching, eczema, psoriasis, neurodermatitis and other skin diseases including cancer.

In the 1950s, two Russian scientists used Aloe Vera extract (sap) for the treatment of periodontal (gum) disease. One hundred and fifty patients were treated by injecting extract at the site of each affected tooth. This treatment completely eliminated periodontal disease in most if not all patients. The research concluded that Aloe Vera is a biogenic stimulator.

Also at about this time Aloe Vera emulsion (sap and gel mixed with mineral oil) was used to treat peptic ulcers in patients for whom long-term conventional therapy offered little or no benefit. Each patient was given a daily dose of Aloe Vera emulsion orally. Researchers reported that 17 of the 18 patients completely recovered from all symptoms of peptic ulcers. The 18th patient left the study after the first dose without any follow-up, so no data was available.

In the 1960s Dr Bill Coates, a pharmacist from Dallas, Texas, discovered a method to extract and stabilise the 'gel' from the leaves using a process that retained the full potency of this amazing healing plant.

By the late 1960s, further dental-related disorders were treated with Aloe Vera. It was found that Aloe Vera had a significant effect in killing or controlling various micro-organisms and concluded that it was a very powerful anti-inflammatory.

In the 1970s, Egyptian researchers wrote of using Aloe Vera (a combination of sap and gel) to treat seborrhoea, acne, alopecia and chronic leg ulcers. They said that Aloe Vera was highly effective against all the above skin problems. Except for studies on peptic ulcers and dental problems, most of the work until this time centred on Aloe Vera's ability to cure skin problems. But it was discovered that Aloe Vera was also a powerful painkiller. At a Chicago burn centre in 1980, it was concluded that the healing effects of Aloe Vera were due to steroidal-like compounds (acting like cortisone) and salicylic acid. It was further stated that, unbelievably, the Aloe Vera completely regenerated hair follicles and allowed for re-growth of hair in burned areas and the presence of salicylic acid in Aloe Vera was reconfirmed. This is an aspirin-like compound, which explains why Aloe helps control pain.

In the 1980s, The National Aloe Science Council (NASC) reported to the FDA that it had developed a standard chemical fingerprint for Aloe Vera. It petitioned the FDA to set US standards for Aloe juice drink, Aloe gel, and other topical products that claim to contain Aloe juice or gel. However, the NASC standard was rejected by the FDA.

Far from stopping the research into what Aloe Vera could do, scientific studies actually increased. It was suggested that drinking Aloe Vera juice improves protein digestion, helps normalise bowel habit, controls yeast infections, promotes proper balance of digestive bacteria, relieves indigestion, irritable bowel syndrome, colitis, acid stomach, and concluded that Aloe juice has no toxic effects. Aloe Vera was also found to be effective in the treatment of shingles (*herpes zoster*).

But it wasn't until the late 1980s that we began to get into very more controversial areas. A Dr McDaniel from Texas stated, 'Aloe extract may mimic AZT without toxicity'. It was said that Aloe Vera stopped progress of AIDS. There were reports that there was a corresponding drop in antibodies to HIV and the number of free viruses in blood samples. McDaniel further concluded that the Aloe would control or kill many other retroviruses, including the viruses that cause the common cold, measles, mumps, chicken pox, flu and other viral diseases. Another Texan doctor, Terry Pulse, maintained that Aloe Vera juice, when orally administered to 69 AIDS patients daily, caused symptoms to disappear almost completely in 81% of the patients and that patients with the AIDS virus who showed no symptoms of the disease remained free of symptoms.

Wilder and wilder claims were made. In India it was recorded that Aloe Vera had virtually eliminated heart disease, stress-related disorders and diabetes in over 4,700 of the 5,000 patients who were followed for five years. All patients were instructed to take a quantity of fresh Aloe Vera plant and psyllium husk and mix it with wheat flour to make a loaf of bread. Treatment consisted of eating one loaf of Aloe bread per day.

Doctors from King Saud University, Saudi Arabia, stated that the dried sap of the Aloe plant was used in the Arabian Peninsula for its ability to lower the blood glucose in diabetic patients. The paper concluded that

Aloes contain a hypoglycemic agent which lowers the blood glucose.

Researchers from Okinawa, Japan, reported in the Japanese *Journal of Cancer Research* that Aloe contained at least three anti-tumour agents, emodin, mannose and lectin. The researchers concluded that Aloe controls pulmonary carcinogenesis and is effective in the treatment of leukaemia and sarcoma and that it would prevent the development of tumours.

In 1990 a paper was presented in Brussels which stated that Aloe, or a substance extracted from it, is a very effective treatment against HIV-1 and other strains of the virus which causes AIDS. That it keeps infected T-4 cells from reproducing the virus, either kills free virus in the blood or stimulates the individual's immune system to kill the virus or both, it stops the disease AIDS from developing in HIV positive patients and can completely reverse the disease in those with full-blown AIDS, and that some patients become syro-negative (i.e. the virus or antibody to the virus can no longer be found in the blood).

In 1994 the US Food and Drug Administration (FDA) approved Aloe Vera for human testing against HIV, the virus that causes AIDS.

Dr Wendell Winters, University of Texas Health Science Centre, reported that Aloe Vera contains at least 140 substances that control cell growth and division, reduce inflammation, stimulate the growth of white cells and other immune-function cells; that it is a wound healer and infection fighter. Winters calls Aloe Vera 'a pharmacy in a plant'.

But what do we *really* know about Aloe Vera today? It seems to heal wounds faster than other methods, it is a powerful laxative, but does it cure cancer and AIDS? Unfortunately, clinical trials don't appear to back this up although some still claim that the plant is a good anti-cancer agent.

Aloe Vera certainly has a cult following, but it is beginning to be seen not only as a folkloric kitchen remedy passed on from generation to generation, but as having properties that will benefit medical science. There is a considerable body of ongoing research regarding the various components of Aloe Vera, to find out more about its properties and to characterise these components so that more specific research can provide clues to the 'magic' that is attributed to the plant.

Obviously we don't know all the answers, but Aloe Vera has been around for almost 4,000 years and has many staunch believers.

The jury is still out.

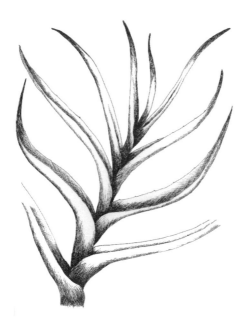

Modern
Miracle or
Ancient Myth?

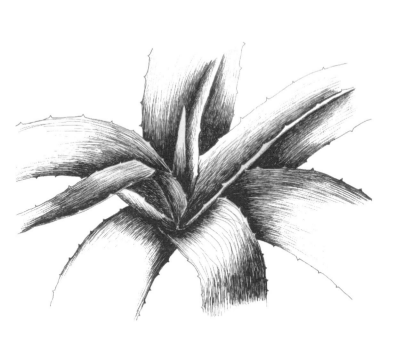

Aloe Vera is not a 'magic bullet' or a 'cure-all'.

The plant has been used since ancient times for healing wounds and burns and treating intestinal problems, such as constipation and worms; in fact the same conditions for which it is still used today.

No wonder the Aloe plant sitting on the kitchen windowsill has served as a favourite multipurpose home remedy throughout history.

But despite the claims of the miraculous properties it possesses, medical science has actually found it to work on just two main areas. The first involves epithelia: epithelial tissue covers the outside of the body (skin) and lines organs and cavities, e.g. sinuses, nose, throat, stomach and bowel. The second is the immune system, which is supposed to protect the body from external invaders such as bacteria, viruses and fungi as well as threats from other foes, such as cancer.

ALOE VERA AND THE EPITHELIUM
Doctors are using Aloe Vera more and more in their practices to treat certain ailments. The more cynical among them may not use Aloe themselves, but will allow their patients to try it, particularly when conventional medicine has failed to alleviate the problem, where there have been side effects from drugs or because patients want to use something more natural.

Aloe Vera gel is used routinely in many burns units in US hospitals. UK doctors have had successes with skin ulcers, acne, eczema, psoriasis, athlete's foot and, surprisingly perhaps, Irritable Bowel Syndrome (IBS).

IBS is not just one ailment, but an umbrella name under which sufferers complain of abdominal bloat, diarrhoea and/or constipation. This is an extremely embarrassing condition, often associated with stress, which can, if it is severe enough, prevent sufferers from going to work or even leaving their homes just in case! It seems so odd that a plant used to alleviate constipation will also help the opposite problem. But in the case of IBS, it is the gel that is used, and for constipation, the remedy is made from the latex.

It must be said again that Aloe Vera gel is not a 'cure', either for skin or digestive illnesses. Many have reported positive results with regular use, but symptoms tend to return after stopping treatment, so taking Aloe Vera needs to be part of an ongoing commitment for the treatment of chronic conditions. Nor does it help everyone, but the failures seem more likely when the stress level is very high.

A trial using Aloe Vera drinking gel for the treatment of ulcerative colitis was carried out at two teaching hospitals in England about six years ago on 44 patients. The conclusion of that trial was that oral Aloe Vera taken for four weeks produces a clinical response more often than with a placebo and appears to be safe. A larger trial involving 200 patients using the same drinking gel was then set up and undertaken in Wales, but the results were inconclusive because not all of the patients responded to the call-back.

THE IMMUNE SYSTEM
With regard to the second quiver in the Aloe Vera bow, people who take Aloe Vera regularly seem to feel generally better. This is probably because the immune system is operating more effectively, keeping colds, coughs, sore throats and flu at bay.

The science of immunology is far too complex to discuss here. Let's just simplify things and say that the immune system works to protect the body from attack. When the immune system is compromised, either from without or within, the sufferer can't fight infection and will surrender to illness or disease. The two most serious instances I can think of are AIDS and peanut allergy. But even healthy people can develop a weakened immune system.

If you think of your immune system as a battleground where there is a constant fight between the 'goodies' and the 'baddies', in a perfect world the 'goodies' fight the battle and triumph and you are none the wiser. When your immune system is weakened, the 'baddies' gain control.

This is where the polysaccharide Acemannan, a major component of Aloe Vera, works. This component acts as an immunomodulator, which means it is able to either step up or slow down the immune response. Polysaccharides are found in every cell in the body and play an important role in lining the colon to prevent absorption of toxins, providing a barrier against microbial invasion, providing lubrication to joints, helping to maintain the level of movement of fluids, allowing the transfer of gases to the lungs and facilitating the absorption of water, electrolytes and nutrients in the gastrointestinal tract.

JUST IN CASE YOU ARE ALLERGIC . . .

Being allergic to Aloe Vera is very rare and it's usually the 'outer skin' rather than the 'inner fillet' that causes the allergic reaction. But like any substance it can be a potential allergen.

Before you use it, there is a simple and easy test you can do at home to find out if you are allergic to Aloe Vera gel. Rub a small amount on your inner arm and wait 24 hours to see if any reaction takes place. If no irritation on the skin is observed then it is generally tolerated. If a burning sensation is experienced wash off with water.

If ingestion causes diarrhoea, reduce the amount you ingest, and slowly increase the amount you ingest over several days until the desired amount is tolerated. Drink plenty of water.

Nature's First Aid Kit:
Aid Kit:

External Uses

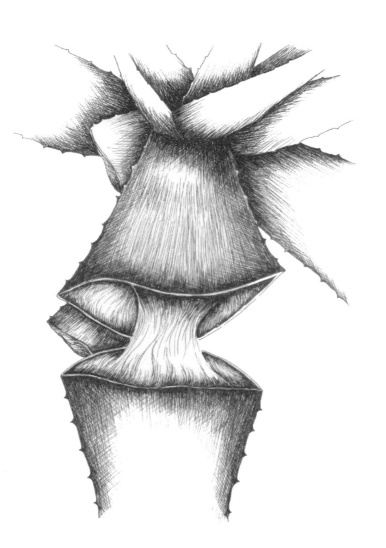

Your skin is the largest organ in your body and it has to last a lifetime, but every day we subject it to torture: scrubbing with soaps, scraping at it with razor blades, using perfumes and colognes that remove moisture from our skin and subjecting ourselves to sun, rain, snow or wind.

So we search for more natural ways to deal with healing, cleansing and moisturising our skin. Externally, Aloe Vera gel has been touted as helpful for a whole alphabet of conditions: abrasions, acne, boils, burns, chafed and cracked skin, cuts and scratches, dandruff, denture sores, insect bites, rashes, psoriasis, stings, sunburn, warts, wrinkles and x-ray burns to name just a few.

Aloe Vera is antibacterial, antiviral and antifungal. Aloe Vera is nature's first aid kit. People have been known to pack small chunks of Aloe Vera gel *inside* wounds that ultimately healed with zero scarring. As the Aloe Vera dries, it actually contracts, pulling the wound shut and keeping it completely free of dangerous bacteria. Plus, it provides nourishment to the wound tissue itself. It's also perfect for use on animals, because if they lick the wound, they won't be licking the toxic chemicals found in most first aid products.

This is not to say that Aloe Vera is going to replace the A & E facility in hospitals. If you have a serious accident and need sutures, you can't just apply Aloe Vera instead of stitches. However, you can use Aloe Vera gel to protect the wound before you set off for the hospital and use it afterwards to aid in the healing process.

If you are involved in outdoor sports, such as hiking, take an Aloe Vera leaf with you. There is quite a lot of gel in a single leaf, so the gel can continue to be used, but since the leaves are not sterile it would be prudent to wrap the cut leaf in clingfilm. It will then continue to be effective for at least a week. It's less cumbersome than carrying a first aid kid and most of what you would have in your kit can be replaced by the Aloe leaf. The severed end of the blade is self-healing. The thin film can easily be broken with each use. Aloe Vera treats cuts, scrapes, burns, bites, stings, punctures, sprains, sunburn and even bruises. And if you are thirsty, with no means of obtaining water, you can eat the gel for its water content.

By placing a protective coating on the affected areas, it accelerates the rate of healing, decreases swelling and redness, increases the availability of oxygen to the skin, increases the strength of tissue, prevents blisters, reduces inflammation and relieves pain. It also aids in keeping the skin supple, draws out infection, helps in the control of acne and eczema, has a moisturising effect on the skin, prevents infection and relieves itching.

Wherever there is damage to epithelial tissue (the inner and outer membranes of the body), Aloe Vera will do its bit to help heal.

Aloe Vera also contains significant levels of salicylic acid (the active ingredient in aspirin) which accounts for some of the plant's pain-killing potential. Some people swear by a burst of aloe spray on sunburn when it is too painful to apply a gel or cream.

ADVANCED WOUND CARE
Carrington Laboratories, located in Irving, Texas, is a major player in research to isolate and stabilise the bioactive ingredients found in the fresh gel of the Aloe Vera plant.

In 1981, Carrington scientists began to search for the unique component of Aloe Vera leaves. In 1982, polymeric mucilaginous polysaccharides were discovered by Carrington. The use of Carrington's stabilised, pharmaceutically prepared gel containing Acemannan Hydrogel™ (a high molecular weight and highly hydrated polymeric mucilaginous polysaccharide) provides the moist wound environment necessary for the natural healing process. It is the only medical device from Aloe Vera distinguished with clearance from the US Food and Drug Administration (FDA) for the management of wounds and cessation of pain.

As the first company to introduce a hydrogel to the wound care market, Carrington has conducted extensive research on the effects of Aloe Vera on wound healing. Below are some of the more common uses of Aloe Vera.

BALDNESS
This theory is rather uncommon, but one Indian internet site, *The Harmony for Silvers Foundation*, a non-government organisation working to enhance the quality of life for the elderly in India, states that one of the main causes of hair loss is toxins in the small intestine. Thus toxin removal by Aloe Vera helps repair this problem and the site claims that local application of Aloe Vera gel on the scalp helps create new cells. Wouldn't it be wonderful if it worked? Worth a try, I'd say.

BURNS
Most people already know that Aloe Vera is wonderfully effective against pain, especially the sort of pain you get from burns. If you've ever burned yourself while cooking, barbecuing, ironing, or stoking a fire, you may be familiar with the soothing qualities of the Aloe plant. It is known as a contact healer because not only does it reduce pain, it stimulates healing on the affected area as well. Modern doctors have also used Aloe Vera for radiation burns, sunburn, chemical burns and first degree burns.

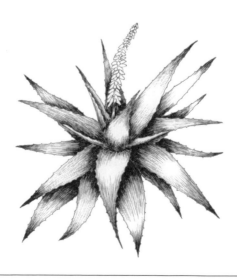

SKIN IRRITATIONS AND CONDITIONS

Aloe Vera is also wonderful for many kinds of skin problems. When applied externally, Aloe Vera gel restores skin tissues. It can also be used on blemishes and for dandruff. One little-known use of Aloe Vera is to relieve itching from chicken pox, poison ivy and poison oak, and to relieve the discomfort of insect bites and stings and the irritation from nettles and other minor skin symptoms. Since it helps remove dead skin and promotes the growth of healthy living cells, it not only causes wounds and burns to heal faster, but it can also improve the general condition of your skin.

ACNE
The type of acne suffered by young people is the result of overactive hormones coupled with bacteria. Technically called *acne vulgaris*, this skin disease affects millions of people annually. It can vary from quite mild to extremely severe. Acne usually develops when the sebaceous glands and the lining of the hair follicle begin to work overtime, as they do in adolescence. Most teenagers have a mild form of this skin problem, which is treatable by consistently applying a non-greasy product such as Aloe Vera gel and keeping the skin and scalp clean.

ECZEMA
Eczema is an inflammation of the skin which can be either sudden or chronic. It is very itchy. Scratching leads to more itching, which leads to more scratching and a vicious cycle is set up. The anti-inflammatory and anti-itch action of Aloe Vera in a moisturising base, such as lanolin, combined with the natural antibiotic bee propolis, is many doctors' treatment of choice.

There might also be some value in drinking Aloe Vera juice at the same time as it will help provide the new skin cells with the micronutrients they need to develop into strong, healthy cells.

PSORIASIS
Psoriasis is a syndrome with a collection of symptoms. It is a disorder of the immune system that may be

hereditary and is exacerbated by stress, alcohol and digestive problems. It can manifest itself as a small, dry flaky patch on the scalp or be much more serious, covering large areas of the body. It is not clear whether Aloe Vera will help this condition, but certainly the topical application of Aloe Vera shampoo, creams and gels will soothe the skin. It is believed that because it is an immune problem, the best treatment is internal, but I would strongly suggest that if you are considering this, you should speak to your doctor first.

It is also said that it might be effective for genital herpes and treating athlete's foot. Aloe Vera gel is also used to shrink warts and lessen the painful effects of shingles. Aloe leaf has also shown outstanding results in treating facial swelling.

HAEMORRHOID RELIEF
Versatile Aloe Vera comes to the rescue once again as a haemorrhoid healer. The very same anti-inflammatory constituents that reduce blistering and inflammation in burns also help reduce the irritation of haemorrhoids. Break off a piece of the aloe vera leaf and apply only the clear gel to the haemorrhoids.

This should help to keep haemorrhoids away and ease the discomfort of a haemorrhoid flare-up. However, don't hesitate to seek your doctor's advice if home remedies aren't enough to get the problem under control.

COSMETICS AND SKINCARE
Used cosmetically, Aloe Vera softens and moisturises the skin. It is especially useful after a warm bath. Because it delivers great results for both skin and hair care, it is common to find Aloe Vera in many types of beauty and cosmetic products. One of the reasons Aloe Vera is so effective is because it can penetrate all three layers of your skin. This can create beneficial results when used with some other all-natural ingredients, such as jojoba oil, which it is often paired with.

Aloe Vera can be used as a cleanser. If a cotton ball is dipped in Aloe gel and applied in an upward and outward motion all over the face, neck and even the areas under and around the eyes, it will help remove dust, grease, oiliness, perspiration, old make-up, etc.

Aloe Vera is also used as an after-waxing relief. The gel is applied over the areas that have been waxed. Aloe helps to soothe, moisturise, heal and cool the waxed skin.

Aloe gel can also be used as an excellent natural aftershave lotion. It can be applied on the shaved areas either by itself or by mixing with a few drops of lime, lavender or rose oil and the gel could even replace shaving cream.

Aloe Vera is very popular for its usage as a shampoo and conditioner. When it comes to hair, it is no secret that the fewer chemicals you expose your hair to, the better it is. Aloe Vera is an excellent natural hair conditioner and can be used in greatly reducing the amount of shampoo you use and can completely eliminate the need to use other chemical conditioners. Some women even use the gel on damp hair instead of over-the-counter hair setting lotions before blow-drying, curling or straightening hair.

Additionally, Aloe Vera gel works on stretch marks, dark circles, spots and blemishes, wrinkles, etc., and is a vital ingredient in the preparation of a great many cosmetic products.

Aloe Vera is included in many over-the-counter lotions, balms, shampoos and sprays. It's really quite amazing how many 'ordinary' products list Aloe Vera as an ingredient. A protective hand cleansing spray that sits on my kitchen sink makes a point of saying it contains Aloe Vera. And looking at the *Household Products Database* published by the National Institutes of Health, just about every popular cosmetic brand lists Aloe Vera as an ingredient. Many of the skin care products containing Aloe Vera are also fortified with vitamin E and collagen to maintain the skin's elasticity and suppleness and keep the moisture in. You can buy suntan lotions containing Aloe Vera. The anti-burning properties of Aloe combined with

SPF factors make it an excellent skin care product. Aloe Vera also has deodorant properties — fresh Aloe along with regular bathing helps control foot odour.

YOUR PETS CAN BENEFIT ALSO!
Aloe Vera is helpful for our dogs and cats, too. The next time your animal companion suffers from a burn, cut or scrape, simply clip off a piece of the fleshy Aloe leaf, slit it open and apply directly to the wound.

Although veterinarians recommend growing your own, you can also buy 100% pure Aloe Vera gel from your local health food store.

Specific Health Benefits and Claims:

Internal Uses

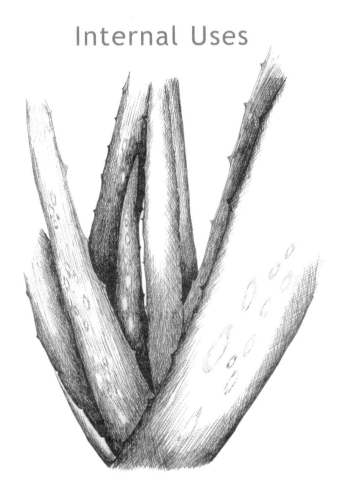

Proponents of Aloe Vera claim that it cures everything from ingrowing toenails to cancer and HIV. Everyone knows someone who has taken Aloe Vera for a medical condition and been helped greatly. There doesn't seem to be any research that says Aloe Vera is harmful to the body, but, on the other hand, a lot of the claims haven't been substantiated . . . yet. And Aloe Vera contains a lot of good stuff! Although many still consider Aloe Vera to be a folk remedy, it is important to remember that two-thirds of the world's population is treated with herbs and plant products that are not only effective, but offer benefits that are equal or superior to the synthesised, chemically derived remedies of the Western world! Plants and herbs have the advantage of causing very few, if any, side effects if they are used properly. Also, there are specific conditions that have responded to herbal treatments when conventional medicine has failed. But Aloe Vera is not just for treating the ill. Healthy people can also benefit.

The primary chemical characteristics of Aloe Vera include aloins, anthraquinones, barbaloin, polysaccharides and salicylic acids. The plant also contains vitamins and minerals including B1, B2, B6 and C, niacinamide, choline, calcium, iron, lecithin, magnesium, manganese, potassium, sodium and zinc. One of the interesting effects of Aloe Vera is that it appears to make vitamin C, vitamin E and other antioxidants work more efficiently. This is probably due to its effect of enhancing blood quality and allowing the blood to transport oxygen and nutrients to the body's cells more effectively.

So it rather sounds as if it could be of great benefit to the system.

If you want to add aloe juice to your diet, start with a small amount, perhaps no more than 60 ml (2 fl oz) a day, and monitor how your body reacts. You can always work up to a higher dosage. For some people, Aloe taken internally can cause cramping and severe discomfort, including loose stools.

ACID REFLUX

Aloe Vera can be very effective in treating acid reflux. Unknown to many, Aloe Vera has the ability to spread a protective coating on the oesophagus and helps in preventing the stomach contents from regurgitating. Taking Aloe Vera may cause diarrhoea in certain people. To avoid this, try taking it with a gas-reducing tea such as peppermint or lemon balm.

BRAIN ACTIVITY

Aloe Vera is said to be very beneficial for the brain. It contains choline which has been shown to boost memory retention. It directly affects nerve signalling and is needed for proper transmission of nerve impulses from the brain through the central nervous system. Other helpful chemicals are boron, phenylalanine, glutamic acid, thiamine and asparagine. They increase mental alertness, neuron activity in the central nervous system, neurotransmitter activity in the brain and spinal cord, aid in detoxifying ammonia out of the brain, optimise cognitive activity and brain function, and also act as an antioxidant and maintain balance in the central nervous system.

CANCER TUMOURS

Dr Lawrence G. Plaskett, a Fellow of the Royal Society of Chemistry, states: 'The action of substances in Aloe Vera does activate and intensify the immune response, and this constitutes one of the fundamental scientifically established actions of Aloe upon the body.'

It is in the boosting of the immune system's response to antigens (foreign elements in the body) that Aloe Vera has shown the most promise in treating cancer. Although no one is yet proposing that Aloe Vera is a *cure* for cancer, it is clear from research conducted throughout the world over the past 30 years that Aloe Vera and, in particular, certain specific substances in the plant have very dramatic and impressive anti-cancer effects. Aloe Vera has been demonstrated to enhance the immune system's response to cancer, promote the growth of new and healthy cells, and reduce the overall viral load within the body thereby revitalising the body in its fight against the disease.

When radiation and chemotherapy are necessary, Aloe Vera helps to minimise the damage done to the body by these treatments, which destroy healthy cells — particularly immune system cells — crucial to the body's recovery. The use of Aloe Vera is said to enable the body to heal itself from cancer and the damage done to it by conventional treatment: the immune system is boosted, tumours shrink, metastases are reduced so the cancer does not spread, and new healthy cells begin to grow.

CHOLESTEROL

When used internally, Aloe Vera gel improves the quality of the blood and helps rebalance the blood chemistry in a way that lowers cholesterol and total triglycerides (in people with elevated levels). Plus, this is far safer than using statins, which can have extremely harmful negative side effects while depleting the body of nutrients such as CoQ10.

I have both heard and read that everyone over the age of 50 ought to be on statins. But, given the possible side effects, those taking statin drugs might strongly consider using high doses of Aloe Vera and blueberries (a powerful antioxidant) to safely wean themselves off the statin drugs (all under the supervision of your GP, of course).

There are natural alternatives that are far safer, less expensive and more effective. Aloe Vera is one of them. An article published in the *British Journal of General Practice* in October 1999 talks about ten studies on Aloe Vera as an aid for reducing blood lipid levels in patients with hyperlipidaemia. Hyperlipidaemia is a condition characterised by increased concentrations of lipids (triglycerides, cholesterol) and lipoproteins (low density lipoproteins (LDL) and very low density lipoproteins (VLDL)) in the blood.

DENTAL USES

Aloe Vera is also used in dental problems such as bleeding gums and denture stomatitis. Stomatitis is an inflammation of the mucous lining of any of the structures in the mouth, which may involve the cheeks, gums, tongue, lips and roof or floor of the mouth. The word 'stomatitis' literally means inflammation of the mouth. The inflammation can be caused by conditions in the mouth itself, such as poor oral hygiene, poorly fitted dentures, mouth burns from hot food or drinks, or by conditions that affect the entire body, such as medications, allergic reactions or infections.

Sprinkle Aloe Vera powder on your toothbrush before brushing. It will help heal gums and whiten your teeth. Drinking Aloe Vera juice also helps heal gums: just swish the liquid around in your mouth a few times before swallowing. Most people with gum disease are also deficient in vitamin D, so if you boost your vitamin D intake as well as treating your gums with Aloe Vera, your results will be greatly accelerated.

DIABETES
It has been suggested that diabetic patients who take Aloe Vera for three months experience a significant drop in fasting blood sugar levels. They also exhibit lower cholesterol levels and slight improvements in total cholesterol. Numerous clinical studies have been published that demonstrate Aloe Vera's anti-diabetic properties.

The same article (mentioned above in Cholesterol) published in the *British Journal of General Practice* suggests that oral administration of Aloe Vera might be a useful adjunct for lowering blood glucose in diabetic patients. Two small, controlled human trials have found that Aloe Vera leaf, either alone or in combination with the oral hypoglycemic drug, glibenclamide, effectively lowers blood sugar in people with type 2 (non-insulin-dependent) diabetes.

Diabetics are also likely to benefit strongly from Aloe Vera's blood enhancements since Aloe reverses 'sludge blood' (the condition that causes blood to form sticky clusters) and boosts circulation to extremities. Diabetics suffering from peripheral neuropathy (hands and feet going numb) are likely to benefit strongly from Aloe Vera supplements.

IBS

Aloe gel is generally considered to be effective in the treatment of IBS, a term used to include a plethora of digestive problems. Irritable Bowel Syndrome is said to affect as many as 12 million people just in Britain alone.

Symptoms include:

- Swollen abdomen
- Unpleasant taste in mouth
- Alternating between diarrhoea and constipation
- A diminished appetite
- Stomach pains that occur low in the abdomen and frequently
- Gas and burping along with a rumbling in the gut in the bowel area
- General feeling of depression and lethargy.
- Heartburn

Polysaccharides in the Aloe Vera plant have curative effects on numerous digestive disorders. The internet is a storehouse of information and testimonials about Aloe Vera curing IBS and other disorders of the digestive tract. This is one of the best-known applications of Aloe Vera gel.

Taking Aloe certainly isn't a magic cure. It won't reverse your disease after drinking one glass of Aloe Vera gel. It needs to be used regularly. Most people report positive results in 3–30 days, depending on the condition. Because Aloe Vera is natural, it works gently within the intestinal tract to help break down food residues that have become impacted and help clean out the bowel. When the bowel is cleaned out, it greatly reduces bloating and discomfort, and helps ease the stress, which only leads to more attacks of Irritable Bowel Syndrome. The sufferer of IBS must begin to watch his or her diet, as there are some foods that are triggers for an attack.

OTHER DIGESTIVE DISORDERS

Aloe Vera juice is said to possess soothing properties that help with colitis, peptic ulcers and digestive tract irritations. Aloe Vera juice contains some anti-inflammatory fatty acids that alkalise digestive juices and prevent over-acidity. European folk medicine makes extensive use of Aloe Vera juice to reduce ulcers and heartburn. Aloe Vera gel is also taken internally for stomach disorders. Dried Aloe latex, another substance derived from the leaf, is a powerful laxative, wellknown for treating severe constipation. It loosens stools, reducing the need to strain when defecating.

If ingestion causes diarrhoea, reduce the amount you drink and slowly increase it over several days until you can tolerate it. Drink plenty of water.

THE IMMUNE SYSTEM
Aloe Vera is rich in mucopolysaccharides, one of which is called Acemannan. Acemannan is being studied for its beneficial effects in boosting T-lymphocyte cells which aid the immune system.

JOINT AND MUSCLE PAIN
Aloe Vera works on joint and muscle pain when used both externally and internally. Essentially, Aloe Vera reduces inflammation. There are many nutritionists who say that if you continue to eat a pro-inflammatory diet that includes red meat, milk, sugar, white flour and fried foods, you will never get rid of inflammation with Aloe alone, but it can help ease the pain while you switch to a healthier way of eating.

WEIGHT LOSS AND MUSCLE DEVELOPMENT
One valuable health benefit for today's society is Aloe Vera's ability to assist weight loss. Aloe Vera works to both reduce and stabilise the body mass index (BMI) by stimulating the metabolic rate in our liver cells so that we burn more energy.

One reason why Aloe Vera works well as a weight loss supplement is because it has a high content of collagen protein. When you drink Aloe Vera juice every day, the body has to spend additional energy to assimilate its protein into your system.

This extra expenditure of energy also supports weight loss and muscle development. Aloe Vera reduces the amount of time food stays in your intestine, which means that less energy is absorbed from the food.

With over 200 nutritional compounds (including vitamin B-12), you should include Aloe Vera juice in any diet/nutrition programme. Aloe Vera alone cannot take the weight off and keep it off. However, Aloe juice twice a day makes sure that you are getting the vitamins and nutrients your body needs as it burns off fat, and builds a lean, toned body. It also facilitates weight loss by helping to expel excess water from the cells.

CONTRAINDICATIONS FOR ALOE VERA

A word of caution: Aloe Vera is contraindicated in pregnant women, breastfeeding mothers, people with garlic and onion allergies and those with kidney problems. Aloe latex will decrease the effectiveness of any medication taken at the same time as it is a laxative and will cause any ingested medication to move through the digestive system too quickly to be effective. If you are on drugs that cause potassium loss or diuretics or steroids, it may not be advisable to take Aloe Vera orally.

This may be overly cautionary, but erring on the side of caution is not a bad thing — some say very small children and little pets should not be given Aloe Vera internally as it can be toxic for them.

Aloe Vera and the Animal World

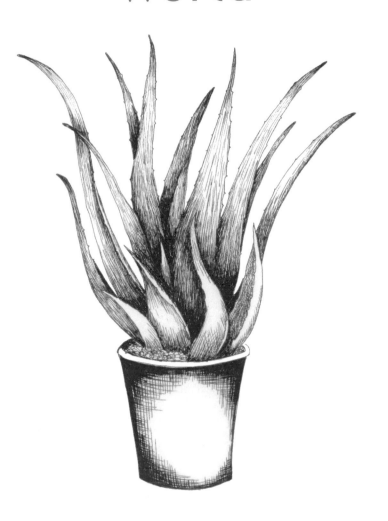

Aloe Vera has been used for centuries for animals as well as people. Most pet owners, farmers and equestrians prefer not to use powerful drugs on their animals because of the unpleasant side effects they may cause. If your animal suffers from skin problems, Aloe Vera may be a better solution because of its proven healing properties.

Aloe Vera is a natural antipruritic — it reduces the itching associated with many skin complaints. Trying to prevent animals from scratching or biting a sore, itchy place is a hopeless task and often requires the animal to wear an itch collar or other device.

Skin products such as Aloe Vera spray, soap, gel and cream can be used to treat pets' inflammatory skin conditions such as dermatitis and eczema, bacterial infections like abscesses, boils and insect bites, and fungal skin complaints, for example ringworm. Wounds made with sharp objects as well as ulcers and burns will also heal more quickly with the use of Aloe Vera. And if you are using a topical Aloe Vera gel to treat your animal and the animal licks it, it will not cause any problems because there aren't any toxic ingredients in it.

The use of Aloe Vera will result in minimum scar formation. It will also cause hair or fur to grow back in its original colour, rather than white, which is a particular consideration for show animals.

Aloe Vera gel can be added to animal feed or drinking water, but cats will probably not like the taste, so if it is painted on the wound instead, the cat will get the benefit of the Aloe by licking it.

More serious diseases have also been treated successfully with Aloe Vera. An injectable form of acemannan, manufactured from Aloe Vera and marketed by Carrington Laboratories as Acemannan Immunostimulant™, has been approved in the USA by the United States Department of Agriculture (USDA) for the treatment of fibrosarcoma (a type of cancer) in dogs and cats after successful clinical trials. In America it is only available through vets.
A similar drug also developed by the same company is being trialled by human HIV sufferers.

An animal doesn't have to be wounded or ill to benefit from Aloe Vera. It can be used as a tonic to grow more lustrous hair and fur, and improve the quality of feathers and skin. Hair, horns and claws are all epithelial tissue. All have been shown to grow faster and more luxuriantly with the addition of Aloe Vera to the animal's diet.

Aloe Vera is not meant to be used as a substitute for conventional veterinary treatment, so please discuss with your vet if your animal is receiving treatment to ensure that Aloe Vera is suitable.

Other
Practical Uses
of Aloe Vera

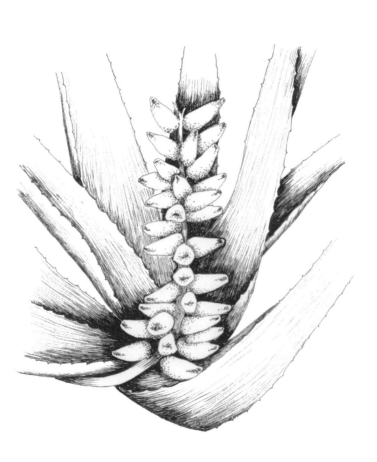

Researchers in Spain have developed an Aloe Vera gel that can be used as an edible coating to prolong the quality and safety of fresh produce.

The gel, which scientists claim does not appear to affect food taste or appearance, could soon provide a safe, natural and environmentally friendly alternative to conventional synthetic preservatives that are currently applied to produce after harvesting.

Researchers at the University of Miguel Hernandez in Alicante, Spain, dipped a bunch of common table grapes into Aloe Vera gel and stored them for five weeks under low temperature while exposing a buch of untreated table grapes to the same conditions.

The colourless Aloe gel used in this study was developed through a special processing technique that maximised the amount of active compounds in the gel.

The untreated grapes appeared to deteriorate rapidly within about seven days, whereas the gel-coated grapes were well-preserved for up to 35 days under the same experimental conditions. The gel-treated grapes were firmer, had less weight loss and less colour change than the untreated grapes, characteristics which correspond to greater freshness.

A sensory panel of ten people evaluated the quality of both the untreated and the gel-treated grapes by consuming some of the grapes. They found that the gel-treated grapes were generally superior in taste.

The Spanish scientists applied for patents at the end of 2005 and it is expected that Aloe Vera gel will be cleared by regulatory bodies in Europe and the USA for commercial use. There are edible coatings used now, some of which contain Aloe Vera, but this is the first time Aloe Vera gel has been used on its own as far as we know. Some of the waxes currently used contain glutens.

The Spaniards didn't assess the added benefit gained from ingesting the Aloe Vera gel coating when eating the fruit but this must be a plus.

In the long term this application method may become available to growers everywhere.

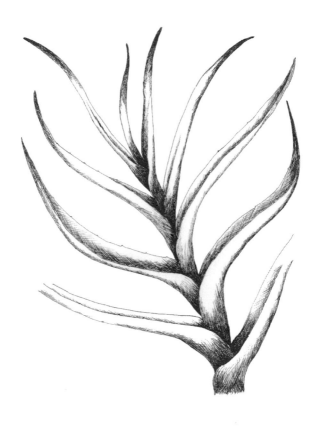

Why Aloe Vera Works

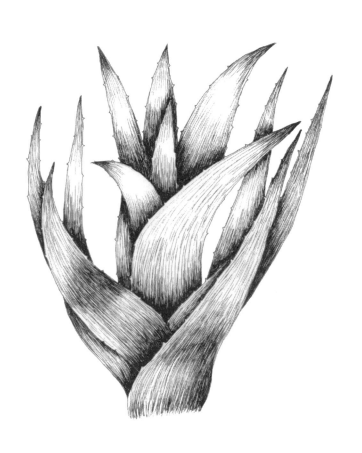

It is surprising that the evident healing effects of Aloe Vera can be produced by such a small quantity of solid factual material. Some people believe that there is a synergistic action between all the component ingredients, giving a result that is greater than the sum of the individual actions.

In orthodox medicine, the practice is to isolate the biologically active substance of the constituent ingredients. These extracted drugs must be uniform in their composition in order to demonstrate a consistent physiological effect. Perhaps there is some truth in an ancient Ayurvedic text from India: 'Extracting drugs from a part of the plant is taking out the intelligence and throwing away the wisdom.' Whole plant preparations, though less potent, are generally considered to be safer, with fewer side effects.

It could be said that Aloe Vera works because the plant produces at least six antiseptic agents: lupeol, salicylic acid, urea nitrogen, cinnamonic acid, phenols and sulphur. All of these substances are recognised as antiseptics because they either kill or control mould, bacteria, fungus and viruses, explaining why the plant has the ability to eliminate many internal and external conditions. The lupeol, a triterpene present in fruits and vegetables, and salicylic acid in the gel explain why it is a very effective painkiller.

Aloe Vera contains at least three anti-inflammatory fatty acids — cholesterol, campersterol and beta-sitosterol (plant sterols), which explains why it is a highly effective treatment for burns, cuts, scrapes, abrasions, allergic reactions, rheumatoid arthritis, rheumatic fever, acid indigestion, ulcers, plus many inflammatory conditions of the digestive system and other internal organs. Beta-sitosterol is also a powerful cholesterol reducer, helping to explain its benefits to heart patients.

Aloe Vera also contains at least 23 polypeptides (immune stimulators), which is why Aloe Vera helps to control a broad spectrum of immune system disorders.

Then there are the amino acids — the building blocks of Aloe Vera.

Amino acids are the basic building blocks of proteins in the production of muscle tissue. Essential amino acids are those that cannot be manufactured by the human body and are essential to the human diet. Aloe Vera contains seven of the eight essential amino acids: isoleucine, leucine, lysine, methionine, phenylalanine, threonine and valine.

Besides building cells and repairing tissue, they form antibodies to combat invading bacteria and viruses; they are part of the enzyme and hormonal system; they build nucleoproteins (RNA and DNA), and they carry oxygen throughout the body and participate in muscle activity. When protein is broken down by digestion the result is (depending on whose research you read) between 20 and 22 known amino acids. These include the essential amino acids above, plus another 12, classified as non-essential, or, in other words, those that can be manufactured by the body with proper nutrition.

The 12 'non-essential' amino acids contained in Aloe Vera are: alanine, arginine, asparagine, cysteine, glutamic acid, glycine, histidine, proline, serine, tyrosine, glutamine and aspartic acid.

The missing 'essential' amino acid is tryptophan, a natural relaxant, which some researchers today actually claim *is* among the amino acids contained in Aloe Vera. Either way 19 out of 20 is a pretty good score!

The evidence suggests that the primary sites of action for Aloe Vera are:

- Epithelial tissues — the epithelium is the layer of cells that covers the surface of the body or lines a cavity that communicates with the surface. The skin, the largest organ of the body, is also the largest epithelial surface — but other epithelial tissues line the nose, sinuses, lungs, mouth, oesophagus and alimentary tract, as well as the genital tract. This action on surfaces and membranes may account for some of the healing properties of Aloe Vera (Davis et al. 1987, Fulton 1990, Heggers 1996).

- The immune system — here, Aloe Vera exerts an effect on the cytokine system, resulting in immunomodulation (Green 1996, Marshall et al. 1993, Winters 1993). It is currently being trialled in human retroviral infection (AIDS).

But after all the theoretical science, Aloe Vera appears to have three very important properties.

IT KILLS BACTERIA, VIRUSES, FUNGI AND YEASTS

At normal strength, good-quality commercial Aloe Vera or material taken from the plant can either destroy or inhibit the growth of several bacterial organisms, especially those that cause skin and wound infections.

From about 1968 to 1972 two doctors in the USA tested stabilised Aloe Vera in an 85% solution against the fungi that causes athlete's foot, which can affect both toe- and fingernails. Further testing in an 80% concentration showed it to work on herpes viruses, including shingles.

In the same 80% concentration, it had good results on persistent yeast infections such as trichomonas and candida.

IT REDUCES INFLAMMATION

Healthy body tissue responds to injury by becoming inflamed. In short, the blood clots, the body attacks invading organisms and healing starts.

However, in certain cases, if one has a hypersensitive allergy, or if the body's tissues are attacked by the inflammation, instead of healing, further tissue damage may occur and the original problem becomes aggravated. These conditions are often treated with non-steroidal anti-inflammatory synthetic drugs, such as ibuprofen. But while this type of drug is effective in reducing symptoms, it can produce unpleasant side effects, such as ulcers or worse.

Aloe Vera is a natural anti-inflammatory agent that works without producing nasty side effects.

IT PROVIDES ESSENTIAL MICRONUTRIENTS
Body tissue (such as skin and intestinal lining) dies and is renewed throughout our lives, but we need a good supply of building materials to produce and maintain healthy and efficient cells. A good diet, rich in key elements, will produce a fit and healthy body and mind. Good nutrition leads to good health.

Eating junk food, however, will result in deficiencies which may lead to disease, so allowing our children to rely on junk food will contribute to a generation of unhealthy adults. Conversely, many diseases can be treated effectively by changes in diet, rather than drugs, which often just treat the symptoms, not the cause.

Aloe Vera appears to have the ability or the potential to heal, alleviate, eliminate or even cure a monumental list of human and animal diseases and disorders.

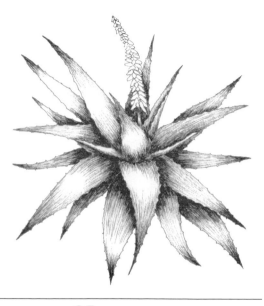

The Future of
Aloe Vera

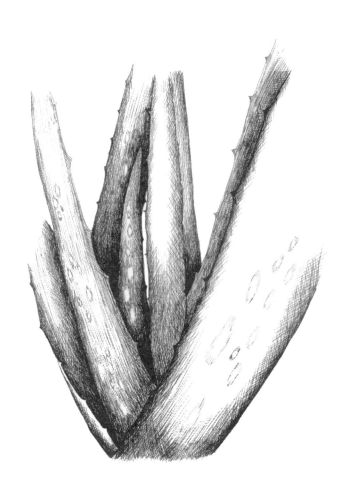

Aloe Vera is starting to be taken seriously, not only by the general public, but by health food companies, cosmetic firms and last, but certainly not least, the medical profession.

Recent uses of Aloe Vera in the medical profession include optometry (there are Aloe eye drops), dentistry (Aloe toothpaste helps inhibit the growth of plaque), Dermatology (Aloe ranks high as an anti-inflammatory agent), gastroenterology (it may be useful in treating chronic inflammation of the digestive system), and perhaps the most recent and exciting area: immuno-depressive disorders, wherein medical science is utilising Aloe Vera for the treatment of the immune system when it is no longer functioning at its optimum capacity.

Health food companies are selling Aloe Vera juice drinks, shampoo and conditioner, gel and gel capsules, one-a-day tablets, toothpaste, colon cleanse tablets, and many more products containing Aloe Vera.

Cosmetic firms, not to be outdone, have added Aloe Vera to shampoo, lipstick, shower gels and aftershave products, citing its moisturising and anti-ageing properties.

Household products such as loo paper, paper tissues and laundry products also proudly declare the addition of Aloe Vera as a soothing additive, and mouthwashes, babies' nappies and women's tights have also had Aloe Vera added to their formulations.

Beauty therapists have discovered the virtues of Aloe Vera gel when used after hair waxing, and hairdressers have found it useful to apply around the hairline before applying hair dye. There are probably many more applications that I haven't even heard of.

But perhaps Aloe Vera's future lies in its clinical application. Many physicians and surgeons have accepted it and it is currently being used in several British hospitals to treat skin conditions and to prevent pain, bruising and burning.

It has also been clinically trialled on a small scale in California. Dr Jeff Bland, a nutritionist, studied the effects of Aloe Vera juice on the GI (gastrointestinal) tract on ten volunteers in 1985. He found improved bowel regularity, increased protein absorption, decreased unfriendly bacteria and yeast, and increased water content of the stool. In this study the use of Aloe also resulted in an overall improvement in an individual's energy and sense of well-being, in addition to enhanced bowel functioning.

Much more recently in Britain, Dr. Peter Atherton, a GP who now writes and lectures about Aloe Vera internationally, was involved in a trial with Professor David Rampton involving 44 people with ulcerative colitis. The conclusion was that oral Aloe Vera taken for four weeks produced a clinical response more often than with a placebo, improved histological (tissue) disease activity, and appeared to be safe.

Another larger trial in Swansea, Wales, using the same drinking gel in the treatment of irritable bowel syndrome, however, proved inconclusive.

Aloe Vera is picking up a large following. It is thought to be an important supplement during this era in history when everyone is considering the benefits of complementary and alternative medicine. We are told we should be responsible for our own health and that we should look after ourselves in terms of diet and fitness and that we should be mindful of the perils of pollutants.

Traditions and Legends

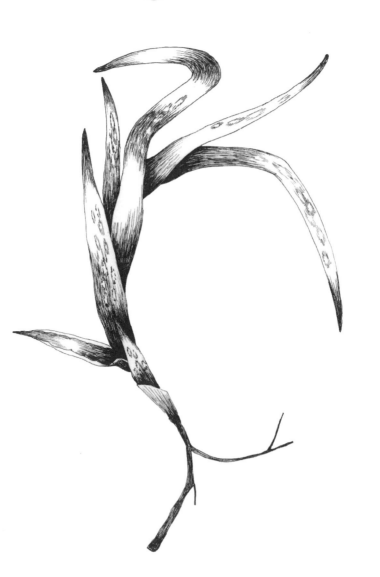

Aloe Vera, called 'nature's miracle' by many, has been associated with myth, magic and medicine since pre-biblical times. All over the world today, Aloe Vera is a common household plant. It is one of the most talked about, yet most misunderstood, plants in history.

Some of its more fanciful applications are to keep a pot in the kitchen to guard against evil spirits, help prevent burns and other mishaps while cooking and to prevent household accidents in general.

Aloe (but probably not the Vera variety) is mentioned in the Bible. '*I have perfumed my bed with myrrh, aloes and cinnamon*' (Proverbs 7:17). For more than 3,500 years, healers and physicians have touted the benefits of this fragrant desert lily. There are about 200 species of aloe, but Aloe Vera, meaning 'true aloe' in Latin, is considered the most effective healer.

The Aloe originates from tropical Africa, where related species are used as an antidote to poison arrow wounds.

According to African folklore, many tribes required everybody in the village to bathe in an infusion of Aloe in case of an epidemic of colds.

African hunters would sometimes rub Aloe Vera juice on their bodies to reduce sweating and mask human body odour.

Aloe Vera was hung above doors of new African homes as a symbol of hope and good fortune.

In Africa today, people still pack whole Aloe leaves around their wounds.

It is believed that the pharaohs and the royal family of Egypt kept Aloe as a palace plant, assigning it a very high status.

Myths and legends surrounding the use of Aloe Vera in ancient times also suggest that it was an important part of the beauty regime of the Egyptian queens Nefertiti and

Cleopatra. Queen Cleopatra regarded the gel as a fountain of youth and used it to preserve her skin against the ravages of time and the Egyptian sun.

The Egyptians were also believed to have used the Aloe plant in their embalming process.

The women of ancient Egypt also believed that the part of Aloe Vera containing aloin caused miscarriages. While it has mostly been proved that this is not true, the myth persists and for that reason, pregnant women are advised against taking Aloe Vera.

It was known to Greeks and Romans, who also used the gel for wounds; one of Pliny's many recommendations was to rub leaves on 'ulcerated male genitals.'

Aloe has been used for at least 2,000 years by the Chinese, who call Aloe Vera 'Lu Hui'. In China, similar uses developed to those in the West, although only the gel is used. Herbs still play a very important part in medicine in China. Today it is used against radiation burns, thermal burns, chapped and dry skin, leg ulcers, skin disorders, as a laxative, to treat burns in general, to help heal disorders of the stomach, liver and spleen, and to expel intestinal worms.

In Indian Ayurvedic medicine Aloe Vera or 'Kumari' is considered one of the most valuable Ayurvedic plants, It has been used to treat a variety of ailments, such as bowel disorders and skin problems, with the gel being a highly regarded cooling tonic for excess 'pitta' (fire element).

Aloe was a favourite purgative during the Middle Ages. Aloe Vera was introduced in Jamaica from West Africa. This medicinal plant is commonly known in Jamaica as 'sinkle bible' and appears in many books about Jamaica and by Jamaicans with that name.

In South America, mothers coat the arms and legs of children with Aloe Vera to keep biting insects away.

In the East Indies, Aloes are used as a varnish to preserve wood from worms and other insects, and to protect skins from insect bites; even living animals are anointed with it for the same reason. The havoc committed by the white ants in India first prompted the trial of Aloe juice to protect wood from them; for which purpose the juice is either used as an extract or in solution with a solvent.

Aloes have been found effective in preserving ships from the ravages of worms and barnacles. The resinous part of this juice is not soluble in water so the ship's bottom, for this purpose, is smeared with a mixture of hepatic aloes (liverleaf), turpentine, tallow and white lead in equal parts. To prove the efficacy of this method, two planks of equal thickness and cut from the same tree were placed under water; one in its natural state, and the other smeared with the mixture. On removal from the water, after being immersed for eight months, the latter was found to be in perfect condition, while the former was entirely riddled with insects and completely rotten.

In Mexico, Aloe Vera plants were placed close to the front door of homes to ensure that those who passed through would have only good intentions.

And in other countries, people would wrap Aloe Vera in paper and give it to newly-weds, without either planting or watering it. If the plant survived, the couple were supposed to have good luck. If it died, I suppose the opposite was assumed.

Closer to home, mothers have been known to stop their children from biting their nails by painting them with the aloin from Aloe Vera.

Aloe Vera is called by many names in many countries but the Japanese 'isha irazu' is the best of all, translating as 'no doctor is needed'.

One of the most famous quotations about Aloe comes from Christopher Columbus:

> Four vegetables are essential to a man's health: wheat, grapes, olives and Aloe. The first is a nutrient, the second fortifies the spirit, the third brings harmony, and the fourth heals.

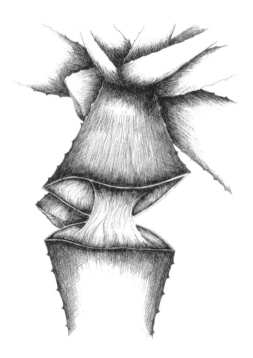

Skincare
Recipes

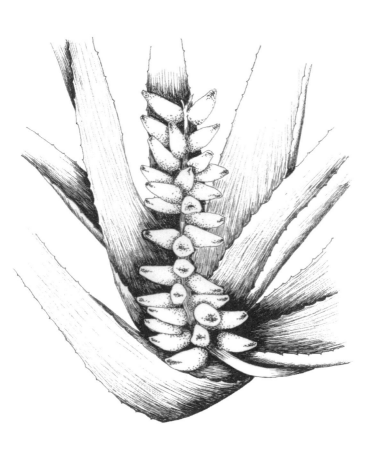

You can make many skincare products for yourself. Why would you want to do this when there are so many skincare products available to buy?

The beauty and skincare market makes many claims to promote their products: for example, the fear of ageing causes us to spend lots of money so that we can look younger, sexier and more desirable. Commercial skin creams are not only expensive, but they can contain long lists of synthetic ingredients. Simple, natural, plant-based creams will do the same job at a fraction of the price and you will have the advantage of knowing what you are using on your skin.

Keep the recipes simple. The less complicated your skincare regime, the better.

Sterilise and dry all equipment and containers, and either wear disposable gloves or make sure you have very clean hands.

You will need the following equipment:

- **JARS AND BOTTLES**
  It is best to have a variety of shapes and sizes of jars and bottles available and glass is definitely better than plastic as you can sterilise it at a high temperature after use and recycle the containers. But I hear that some companies now offer sterilised plastic containers, which is safer if you are using the products in your bathroom. Jars and bottles are available from a number of sources on the internet and from some speciality craft shops.

- **GLASS MIXING BOWL AND GLASS ROD**
  A glass mixing bowl or jug and a glass rod are best for blending these products as they can be properly sterilised after use. If you don't have a glass rod, a metal spoon can be used instead.

Since you are not adding preservatives, for greatest safety freeze the formulas in small portions and thaw out what you need when you need it.

If anything doesn't smell quite right to you or if the odour changes, discard it.

Apply a small amount of your chosen recipe with damp hands or just after bathing to keep your skin soft and protected. If an oil is called for in a given recipe, for younger skin try apricot kernel oil, coconut oil, hemp seed oil, wheatgerm oil or olive oil. More mature skins will benefit from avocado oil or evening primrose oil. For all skin types, almond oil, jojoba oil or cocoa butter are good choices.

For all the skin recipes using Aloe Vera gel, you can either use the colourless gel from a cut leaf of an Aloe Vera plant or 100% pure Aloe Vera gel purchased from a health food or beauty shop. Avoid the yellow latex liquid, found near the surface of the leaf. This liquid, called aloin, is not suitable for skincare.

ALWAYS DO A PATCH TEST BEFORE USING ANY HOMEMADE BEAUTY RECIPES.

Allergic reactions to Aloe Vera gel are very rare and it's usually the latex or aloin that causes the reaction rather than the gel. But like any other substance, it has the potential to be an allergen.

Before you use it, there is a simple and easy test you can do at home to find out if you are allergic to Aloe Vera gel. Rub a small amount on your inner arm and wait 24 hours to see if any reaction takes place. If no irritation on the skin is observed, then it is generally tolerated. If a burning sensation is experienced, wash off with water.

SOAPS AND CLEANSERS

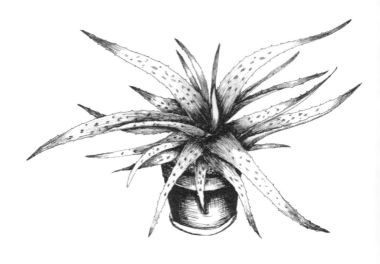

ALOE AND NETTLE SOAP

You will need:

240 ml (8 fl oz) glycerine soap base
30 ml (2 tbsp) Aloe Vera gel
30 ml (2 tbsp) powdered nettle leaf or nettle leaf extract

Method:

1. Microwave the glycerine soap base in a glass measuring cup until melted.
2. Mix in the Aloe Vera and nettle, pour into soap moulds and cool.

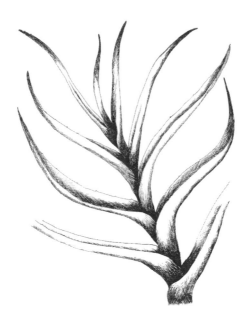

ALOE SOAP BALLS

You will need:

115 g (4 oz) grated mild soap
30 drops evening primrose oil
30 ml (2 tbsp) Aloe Vera gel
25 ml (1½ tbsp) rosewater
10 drops essential oil of your choice
1 drop candle or soap colouring (optional)

Method:

1. Mix the grated soap with the evening primrose oil,
Aloe Vera and rosewater. Cover and let stand overnight.
2. Put the mixture into a food processor, and blend with
the essential oil and add food colouring if using.
3. Moisten your hands and form the mixture into balls.
4. Place on greaseproof paper to dry.
5. Store in a glass or plastic container.

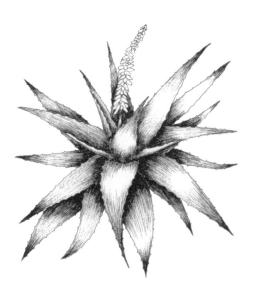

CUCUMBER LOOFAH SOAP

This natural hand-made recipe creates a soap that gives your skin a natural and healthy glow. The ground loofah flakes act as a gentle exfoliator.

It is easy to make natural handmade soap products. Feel free to substitute or add fragrance oils, herbs or salts to personalise your natural handmade recipes.

It is also a great gift idea. Your friends and family will appreciate the gift of a relaxing and unique bath and body product.

Presentation plays an important role in the gift-giving of your handmade soaps, salts and lotions. Below are several packaging ideas, but don't let this brief list limit your creativity!

Paper is a popular packaging medium because of the variety of papers available. You can use brown wrapping paper, marbled paper, gift wrap, wallpaper, newspaper, tissue paper or anything else that strikes your fancy. Your creativity is the limit! You can use your computer to add designs and logos to plain paper or you can paint or draw on the paper for an added personal touch. When wrapping soap, you can wrap individual bars and either leave plain or add extra embellishments by tying with ribbons, cord, raffia or lace.

Boxes and baskets are nice containers for soap, especially when you fill the boxes with other materials. You can fill the box or basket halfway with herbs, dried flowers or pot-pourri that match the scent of your soap. Gift basket fillings, other toiletries, face cloths or sponges also make great fillers in the basket with your loofah soap. Once you have added the filler and soap, wrap the box or basket in cellophane or tissue paper.

You will need:

Loofah (natural sponge)
Soap moulds
85 g (3 oz) mild fragrance-free soap
120 ml (4 fl oz) distilled or filtered water
15 ml (1 tbsp) Aloe Vera gel
10 ml (2 tsp) ground loofah flakes
15 drops cucumber fragrance oil
Green food colouring (optional)

Method:

1. Slice the loofah thinly to the size of your moulds and put one slice in each mould.
2. Shred the soap in a food processor.
3. Place the water over a low heat and stir in the shredded soap. Continue stirring until the mix becomes a sticky mass, which will take approximately 4 minutes. Remove from the heat and stir in the Aloe Vera gel, the ground loofah flakes, the cucumber fragrance oil and the food colouring (if using) until well blended. Spoon the mixture into the moulds containing the loofah slice and allow it to set for 6 hours until hardened.

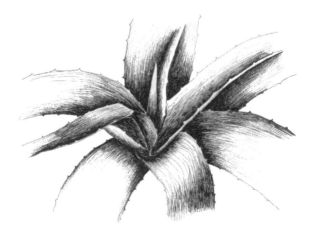

LEMON ALOE CLEANSER FOR OILY SKIN

You will need: **Makes about 200 ml (7 fl oz)**

60 ml (4 tbsp) porridge oats
30 ml (2 tbsp) maize meal
30 ml (2 tbsp) grated lemon rind
10 ml (2 tsp) Aloe Vera gel
30 ml (2 tbsp) lemon pulp and juice
60 ml (4 tbsp) plain yogurt

Method:

1. Process the porridge oats into a powder in a blender or spice grinder.
2. In a small bowl, mix the oats with the maize meal and lemon rind.
3. Add the Aloe Vera gel, lemon pulp and juice and yogurt and whisk until creamy in texture. Scoop into a cosmetic jar or squeeze bottle and store in the refrigerator for up to one month.
4. Spread over oily areas of your face, massaging gently for up to 10 minutes using a circular motion. Avoid the area around your eyes and lips.
5. Rinse well with warm water.
6. Apply toner and moisturiser.

Note: This cleanser may be used 2–3 times a week if necessary, but if you are going out in the sun, cleanse afterwards as the astringent lemon may cause sunburn.

VITAMIN E SOAP

You will need:

60 ml (4 tbsp) 100% Aloe Vera gel
200 ml (7 fl oz) mineral, spring or filtered water
340 g (12 oz) grated pure soap
30 ml (2 tbsp) vitamin E base oil
1 drop green candle and soap colouring (optional)

Method:

1. Put the Aloe Vera gel and water into a saucepan and add the grated soap.
2. Heat gently until the soap is melted.
3. Remove from the heat and add the vitamin E oil and soap colour if using.
4. Pour into soap moulds and set aside to solidify.

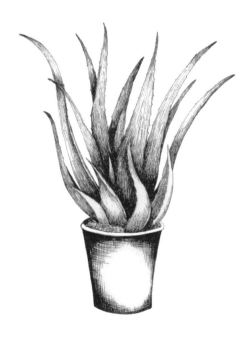

EMPRESS JOSEPHINE'S
CLEAR COMPLEXION CLEANSER

Josephine de Beaubarnais married Napoleon Bonaparte in 1796. The Empress was well-known for her beautiful, clear complexion. This is the cleanser she is supposed to have used.

You will need: **Makes 150 ml (5 fl oz)**

    120 ml (4 fl oz) Aloe Vera gel
    30 ml (2 tbsp) fresh whole milk

Method:

1. Mix the Aloe Vera and milk together until smooth.
2. To use, pour a small amount into your palm and massage gently onto your face.
3. Rinse well and pat dry.
4. Store in a suitable cosmetic container in the refrigerator. Smell before using as milk turns sour.

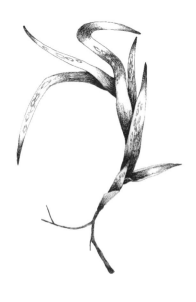

FACIAL MOISTURISERS AND MASKS

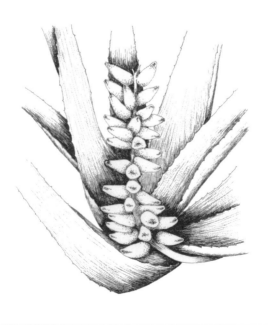

A RELAXING FACIAL MASK

Cosmetic clays (or natural silicates) are the single most perfect base materials for facial masks. They stimulate circulation by generating heat as they dry and promote toxin elimination (impurities are drawn out of the skin's tissues like a magnet, binding to the clay minerals). Clays are excellent for inflamed skin, because they restore it to its proper equilibrium. Clays are perfectly safe, but can tend to dry skin if used too often. We suggest no more than once a week.

THE BASIC FACIAL MASK

Easy to prepare, effective, and wonderfully relaxing.

You will need:

A non-metallic bowl (glass is best)
A non-metallic spoon (wood is fine)
Distilled water, spring water, or floral water (this is best)
Cosmetic clay, e.g. French white clay
Essential oils, fruit juice, etc. (optional)

Method:

1. Sprinkle equal amounts of clay and distilled water (or other liquid) into bowl.
2. Mix until a soft paste is obtained.
3. Let stand for several minutes so that the clay absorbs all the water.
4. Add any other desired ingredients (depending on your skin type), such as essential oils, etc.
5. If the preparation is too liquid, add more clay – if too solid, add more water.
6. Apply to the skin, covering the whole face except for the eyes and mouth area.
7. Soak a cotton pad in water with 1–2 drops of German (blue) chamomile and place over eyes, or place a thick cucumber slice over each eyelid.

8. Lie back and relax with feet elevated on a soft pillow (or place the pillow under your knees).
9. Allow 15–20 minutes for the clay to completely dry (as long as the clay is wet, it is still working).
10. Rinse with warm water and pat dry.
11. Follow with a spray of floral water.

Variations for specific skin types:

NORMAL SKIN:
Use either Moroccan red or rose clay mixture (a combination of Moroccan red and French white clay). Try adding puréed cucumber or a little puréed avocado to the mix. Instead of water, try lavender, rose, rose geranium or chamomile floral water (these are appropriate for all skin types). For a particularly effective liquid, combine 2 parts sparkling mineral water, 2 parts floral water and 1 part Aloe Vera gel. To the prepared paste, you might also add a few drops of hazelnut, jojoba, avocado or almond oil and a few drops of lavender, rose geranium or chamomile essential oil.

SENSITIVE SKIN:
Calendula oil, natural honey and Aloe Vera gel can be added to the paste. Rose, neroli and chamomile are excellent essential oils for sensitive skin, too.

ALOE AND HONEY FACIAL MASK

(FOR ALL SKIN TYPES)

The combination of Aloe Vera's soothing properties and honey's gentle astringent and hydrating benefits make this a perfect treatment for any time of the year.

You will need: **Makes enough for one treatment**

    5 ml (1 tsp) Aloe Vera gel
    5 ml (1 tsp) honey

Method:

1. Mix the Aloe Vera and honey together in a small dish.
2. Apply to the face (being careful not to get it in your eyes) with clean fingers and leave on for 10 minutes.
3. Rinse off with warm water.

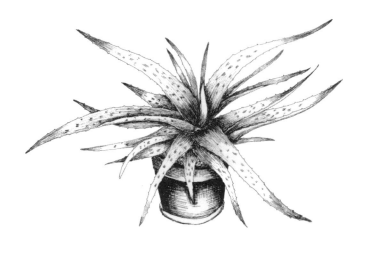

ALOE AND VITAMIN E LOTION

You will need: **Makes about 150 ml (5 fl oz)**

120 ml (4 fl oz) Aloe Vera gel
2.5 ml (½ tsp) lanolin
2.5 ml (½ tsp) vitamin E oil
75 ml (5 tbsp) almond oil
20 g (½ oz) beeswax pellets

Method:

1. In a small blender combine the Aloe Vera gel, lanolin and vitamin E oil together.
2. Microwave the beeswax and almond oil in a small glass beaker until melted.
3. Add the melted beeswax mixture to the blender in a slow stream while blending on low.
4. Once all the beeswax has been added, blend for another 2 or more seconds until the mixture looks like whipped cream.
5. Scoop into a suitable cosmetic pot.

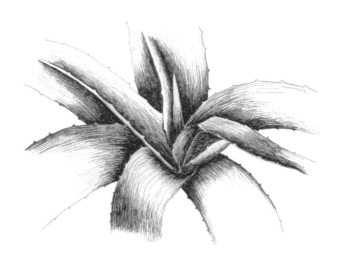

ALOE VERA COLD CREAM

The Aloe Vera adds a wonderful texture to this lovely cleansing and moisturising cream.

You will need: **Makes about 150 ml (5 fl oz)**

    15 ml (1 tbsp) Aloe Vera gel
    75 ml (5 tbsp) olive oil
    15 g (½ oz) beeswax pellets
    30 ml (2 tbsp) lanolin
    2–3 drops rose or lavender essential oil
    30 ml (2 tbsp) rosewater

Method:

1. Using a wire whisk or a blender, mix the Aloe Vera gel into the olive oil. Set aside.
2. Microwave the beeswax with the lanolin in a glass dish until melted, about 30 seconds. Remove from the microwave and stir in the essential oil.
3. Stir in the rosewater and keep stirring until the mixture starts to thicken.
4. Pour into a cosmetic jar and cover tightly.

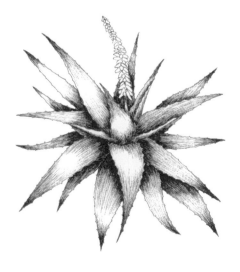

BLUEBERRY ALOE FACIAL MASK

The spirulina, chamomile extract and lavender essential oil can all be purchased from health food stores.

You will need: **Makes enough for one treatment**

2 dried chamomile flower extract capsules
15 ml (1 tbsp) spirulina
5 ml (1 tsp) fresh or frozen blueberries, puréed
60 ml (4 tbsp) Aloe Vera gel
4 drops lavender essential oil

Method:

1. Break the chamomile flower and spirulina capsules into a small bowl. Mix with the blueberry purée and Aloe Vera.
2. Cleanse your face and then steam over a bowl of hot water to open your pores. Apply the mask and leave on for 20 minutes.
3. Remove the mask with a warm, damp face cloth, rinse your face with cool water to close your pores and follow with moisturiser.

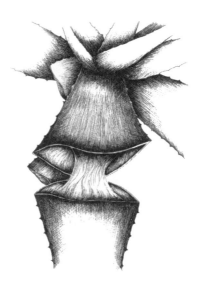

CALENDULA MOISTURISING CREAM

This is a wonderful rich moisturiser that can be used as a day cream for normal to dry skins and as a night cream for all skin types. Since this recipe makes rather a lot of cream, you could share it with your very good friends.

You will need: **Makes 300 ml (10 fl oz)**

45 ml (3 tbsp) coconut oil
30 ml (2 tbsp) apricot kernel oil
30 ml (2 tbsp) grapeseed oil
20 ml (4 tbsp) almond oil
15 ml (1 tbsp) calendula oil
15 g (½ oz) beeswax pellets
2.5 ml (½ tsp) cocoa butter
60 ml (4 tbsp) chamomile tea
90 ml (6 tbsp) distilled water
30 ml (2 tbsp) Aloe Vera gel
Your choice of essential oils

Method:

1. Combine the coconut oil, apricot kernel oil, grapeseed oil, almond oil calendula oil, beeswax pellets and cocoa butter in a small saucepan and melt over a low heat. Remove from the heat immediately when melted. Pour the mixture into a glass measuring cup and allow to cool to room temperature.
2. Pour the tea, distilled water and Aloe Vera gel into a blender (these must also be at room temperature). Turn the blender to its highest speed and very slowly add the cooled oil mixture. Blend until the cream is thick and white. The blender will start to sputter, signalling that the cream has reached the proper consistency. Turn the blender off.
3. If you want to use several different essential oils, pour the cream into glass jars and add essential oils of your choice, in a ratio of 7–10 drops to each 30 ml (1 fl oz) of cream, stirring well. If you want to use the same

essential oil, you can do it at the end of the previous step.

> *Note*: It is important that the temperature of the oils and the waters is the same when you combine them to avoid separation of the cream. However, if separation does occur, just shake before using.

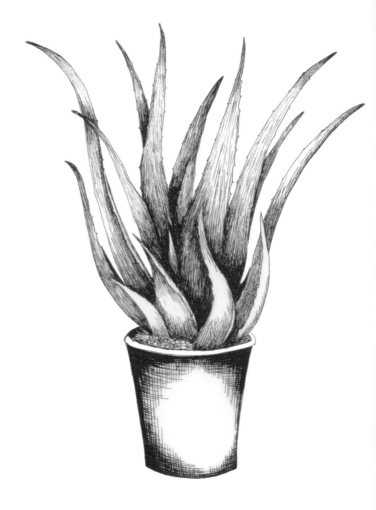

DRY SKIN MOISTURISING CREAM

This cream has marvellous restorative qualities because of the inclusion of Aloe Vera, vitamin E and a variety of oils chosen to give dry, tired skin moisture and radiance.

You will need: **Makes about 550 ml (almost 1 pint)**

180 ml (6 fl oz) olive oil
75 ml (5 tbsp) virgin coconut oil
55 g (2 oz) beeswax pellets
150 ml (5 fl oz) distilled water
75 ml (5 tbsp) Aloe Vera gel
6 drops lavender essential oil
1.25 ml (¼ tsp) vitamin E base oil
3 drops grapeseed extract

Method:

1. Combine the olive oil, coconut oil and beeswax in a microwavable bowl and melt in the microwave.
2. Pour the mixture into a heavy-duty blender or electric mixer and let cool until it is the consistency of double cream.
3. While the olive oil mixture is cooling, combine the water, Aloe Vera, lavender oil, vitamin E oil and grapeseed extract in a large measuring cup.
4. When cool enough, pour the second mixture into the blender or mixer and blend until smooth and creamy. The mixture will be very heavy.
5. Store the cream in small cosmetic jars in the refrigerator.

Note: The oil and water mixtures must be pretty close to the same temperature, or they will not emulsify.

FACIAL MASK FOR OILY SKIN

You will need: **Makes enough for one treatment**

30 ml (2 tbsp) cosmetic clay
5 ml (1 tsp) Aloe Vera juice
2.5 ml (½ tsp) jojoba oil
1 drop bergamot oil
1 drop lavender oil

Method:

1. Mix all the ingredients in a glass bowl with enough water to make a paste.
2. Apply to your face, avoiding the eyes and mouth, and leave on until the clay is dry.
3. Rinse gently with warm water.

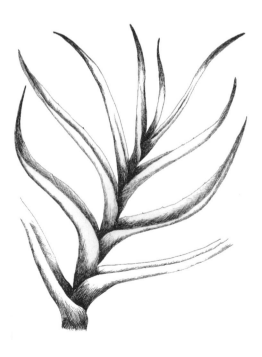

FRESH ROSE MOISTURISER

You will need: **Makes 500 ml (17 fl oz)**

240 ml (8 fl oz) distilled or filtered water
15 g (½ oz) fresh red rose petals
240 ml (8 fl oz) glycerine
15 ml (1 tbsp) Aloe Vera gel

Method:

1. In a small saucepan, heat water and rose petals until just boiling. Let the rosewater cool, then strain out the petals.
2. Pour rosewater into your cosmetic bottle. Then pour in the glycerine and Aloe Vera. Cap the bottle securely and shake well to blend.
3. Store your moisturiser in the refrigerator. Shake gently before each use.
4. Try to avoid getting it in your eyes.

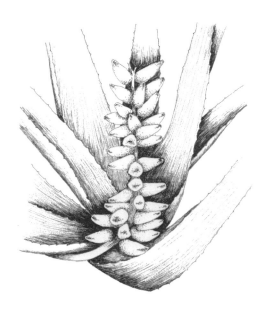

HYDRATING FACIAL MIST

You will need: **Makes 150 ml (5 fl oz)**

    60 ml (4 tbsp) still mineral water
    30 ml (2 tbsp) orange flower water
    30 ml (2 tbsp) rosewater
    30 ml (2 tbsp) Aloe Vera gel

Method:

1. Combine all the ingredients in a cosmetic spray bottle
and shake until well blended.
2. Use as needed, storing the remainder in the
refrigerator.

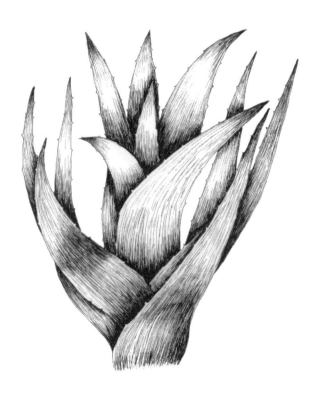

SOOTHING NIGHT CREAM

You will need: **Makes about 100 ml (3½ fl oz)**

45 ml (3 tbsp) olive oil
15 ml (1 tbsp) shea butter
15 g (½ oz) beeswax pellets
1.25 ml (¼ tsp) vitamin E base oil
1.25 ml (¼ tsp) lecithin
15 ml (1 tbsp) rosewater
15 ml (1 tbsp) Aloe Vera gel
3 drops chamomile essential oil

Method:

1. Microwave the olive oil, shea butter and beeswax pellets in a small glass bowl until melted. Remove from the oven just before the beeswax is completely melted. Finish melting by stirring.
2. Add the vitamin E oil and lecithin and stir.
3. Mix the rosewater and Aloe Vera together and slowly add to the oil mixture. Continue stirring with a small metal whisk.
4. Once the mixture is cool, add the chamomile oil. Pour into a suitable container and store in a cool dark place.
5. Use nightly, especially in cold weather or if your skin is very dry.

Note: As in all water—oil mixtures, the waters and the oils must be the same temperature when they are combined to emulsify properly.

BODY LOTIONS AND BUTTERS

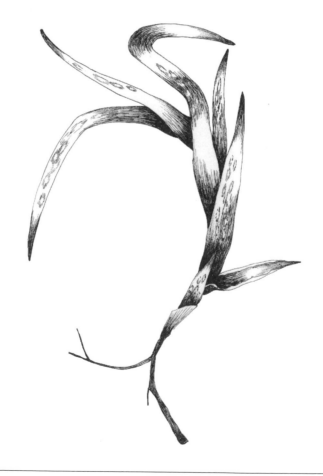

ALOE VERA BODY LOTION

You will need: Makes approximately 480 ml (16 fl oz)

225 g (8 oz) Aloe Vera gel
5 ml (1 tsp) lanolin
5 ml (1 tsp) vitamin E oil
75 ml (5 tbsp) virgin coconut oil
15 g (½ oz) beeswax pellets
180 ml (6 fl oz) almond oil
Up to 7.5 ml (1½ tsp) essential oil of your choice

Method:

1. Place Aloe Vera gel, lanolin and vitamin E oil in a blender or food processor.
2. Place coconut oil and beeswax pellets in a glass measuring cup and microwave on high for 30 seconds, then stir. Repeat in 10-second bursts until fully melted.
3. Remove from the oven. Stir in almond oil, reheating if necessary. Run blender at low to medium speed and then pour in melted oils in a thin stream. As the oils are blended in, the cream will turn white and the blender's motor will begin to slow. As soon as you have a mayonnaise-like consistency, stop the motor, add the essential oils and pulse blend. Do not overblend.
4. Transfer the cream to glass jars while still warm because it thickens quickly.

Note: This recipe does not require refrigeration, but all equipment must be scrupulously clean and free of bacteria. Cleaning with boiling water and surgical spirit is a good way to kill bacteria naturally.

BODY BUTTER

You will need: **Makes about 175 ml (6 fl oz)**

    120 ml (4 fl oz) Aloe Vera gel
    20 ml (4 tsp) cornflour
    15 ml (1 tbsp) witch hazel
    3—4 drops peppermint oil

Method:

1. Mix Aloe Vera, cornflour and witch hazel in a glass bowl.
2. Microwave 1—2 minutes, stirring at 30-second intervals until mixture is clear and thick.
3. Scoop into an appropriate cosmetic container.
4. Use after a bath or shower to keep your skin looking and feeling moist and smooth.

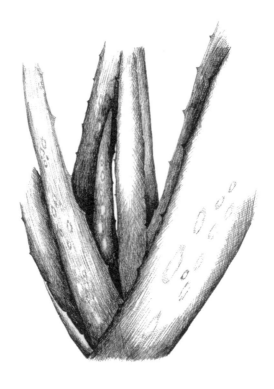

CUCUMBER AND ALOE AFTER-BATH SPRAY

(FOR ALL SKIN TYPES)

You will need: **Makes about 300 ml (10 fl oz)**

  1 cucumber, chopped
  60 ml (4 tbsp) witch hazel
  60 ml (4 tbsp) distilled water
  5 ml (1 tsp) Aloe Vera gel

Method:

1. Whizz the cucumber in a blender, strain the juice and set aside. Discard the cucumber solids.
2. Mix the cucumber juice with the witch hazel, distilled water and Aloe Vera gel and pour into a spray bottle.
3. Spray on to clean skin after bathing or whenever your skin needs a lift. The cool scent will boost your spirits and tone your skin.
4. Store the mixture in the refrigerator and use quickly. This mixture spoils easily.

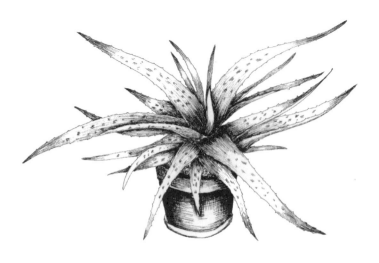

ORANGE ALMOND CREAM

A WONDERFUL ALL-PURPOSE SKIN CREAM

You will need: **Makes about 500 ml (17 fl oz)**

150 ml (5 fl oz) orange flower water
75 ml (5 tbsp) Aloe Vera gel
1–2 drops sweet orange essential oil
1.25 ml (¼ tsp) vitamin E base oil
180 ml (6 fl oz) almond oil
75 ml (5 tbsp) cocoa butter
1.25 ml (¼ tsp) lanolin
15–30g (½–1 oz) beeswax pellets

Method:

1. Combine orange flower water, Aloe Vera gel, essential oil and vitamin E oil in a glass measuring cup. Set aside.
2. In a double boiler over a low heat, combine remaining ingredients. Heat just enough to melt.
3. Pour oils into a blender and let cool to room temperature. The mixture should become thick, creamy, semi-solid and cream-coloured. This cooling process can be hastened in the refrigerator, but keep an eye on it so it doesn't get too hard.
4. When cool, turn blender on the highest speed. Drizzle the water mixture slowly into the blender while it is running.
5. When most of the water mixture has been added to the oils, listen to the blender and watch the cream. When the blender sputters and the mixture looks like butter cream icing, turn off the blender. You can slowly add more water, whisking it in by hand with a spoon, but don't overbeat. The cream will thicken as it sets.
6. Pour into cream or lotion jars and store in a cool place.

JASMINE BODY LOTION

You will need: **Makes 340 ml (12 fl oz)**

150 ml (5 fl oz) distilled water
30 ml (2 tbsp) dried jasmine flowers
15 ml (1 tbsp) Aloe Vera gel
10 ml (2 tsp) vitamin E base oil
10 ml (2 tsp) grapefruit seed extract
60 ml (4 tbsp) grapeseed oil
60 ml (4 tbsp) almond oil
5 ml (1 tsp) shea butter
5 ml (1 tsp) beeswax pellets
1.25 ml (¼ tsp) benzoin essential oil
10 drops jasmine essential oil

Method:

1. First make the jasmine infusion. In a microwave-safe measuring cup heat the water until it is almost boiling. Add the jasmine flowers and let steep for 30 minutes.
2. With a coffee filter set into a funnel over a measuring cup, strain the jasmine mixture to remove the solids. Place the infusion in a heatproof bowl, add the Aloe Vera, vitamin E oil and grapefruit seed extract and set aside.
3. Add the grapeseed oil, almond oil, shea butter and beeswax to a clean microwave-safe glass bowl and heat until the beeswax is melted. Remove from the heat and immediately add the benzoin oil and stir well.
4. Pour the oil mixture into the prepared jasmine infusion and pour into a blender quickly. Keep blending until the mixture becomes opaque and smooth. Add the jasmine oil while you are blending.
5. Pour the lotion into a dark glass cosmetic bottle and place in the refrigerator to cool. Do not put the cap on until the mixture is cold.
6. Apply to damp skin after a shower or bath.
7. Store the unused lotion in the refrigerator.

RICH AND ROSY HAND CREAM

You will need: **Makes about 500 ml (17 fl oz)**

180 ml (6 fl oz) almond oil
45 ml (3 tbsp) virgin coconut oil or cocoa butter
5 ml (1 tsp) lanolin
15 g (½ oz) beeswax pellets
150 ml (5 fl oz) rosewater
120 ml (4 fl oz) Aloe Vera gel
1—2 drops rose fragrance oil
5 drops vitamin E base oil

Method:

1. Melt the first 4 ingredients together in a microwave oven or over a low heat and cool to room temperature.
2. When cool, add the rosewater, Aloe Vera, rose fragrance oil and vitamin E oil.
3. Whip the mixture to a smooth consistency.
4. Store in a sterile covered jar.

LEG AND FOOT CARE

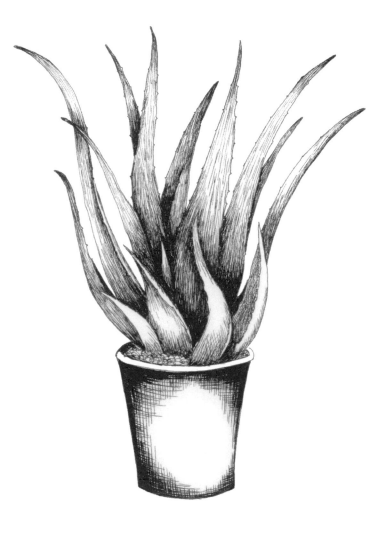

FOOT BALM

You will need: **Makes 50 ml (about 2 fl oz)**

30 ml (2 tbsp) avocado, jojoba, almond or apricot kernel oil
15 g (½ oz) beeswax pellets
1.25 ml (¼ tsp) vitamin E base oil
2.5 ml (½ tsp) Aloe Vera gel
few drops peppermint essential oil

Method:

1. Microwave the oil of your choice with the beeswax in a glass bowl on high for 2 minutes.
2. Remove from the oven when the wax has melted. Add the vitamin E oil, Aloe Vera and peppermint oil and stir well.
3. Pour into a glass or plastic cosmetic container and store in a cool, dark place.
4. Massage into your feet whenever they need pampering.

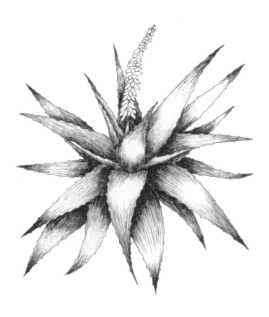

EXFOLIATING FOOT MASK

You will need: **Makes about 500 ml (17 fl oz)**

40 g (1½ oz) porridge oats
85 g (3 oz) maize meal
115 g (4 oz) coarse sea salt
120 ml (4 fl oz) almond oil
60 ml (4 tbsp) Aloe Vera gel

Method:

1. In a food processor or spice grinder, process the porridge oats.
2. Mix all the ingredients together in a large bowl until moistened. If the mixture is too crumbly, add some more almond oil and Aloe Vera.
3. Scoop into a large cosmetic bottle.
4. To use, pour some of the foot mask into a basin and, one foot at a time, put your feet into the basin and massage, beginning with the toes and working up to the heel and ankle. Rinse with warm water and dry, ensuring that you dry well between your toes.
4. Store the excess foot mask in the refrigerator until needed.

COOLING LEG GEL

You will need: **Makes about 150 ml (5 fl oz)**

120 ml (4 fl oz) Aloe Vera gel
7.5 ml (1½ tsp) cornflour
15 ml (1 tbsp) witch hazel
4 drops peppermint essential oil

Method:

1. Combine the Aloe Vera, cornflour and witch hazel in a small glass bowl and microwave until thick and clear for about 2 minutes, stirring at 30-second intervals.
2. Allow to cool and then stir in the peppermint oil.
3. Pour into a cosmetic bottle.
4. To use, massage into legs and feet.

HAIR TREATMENTS

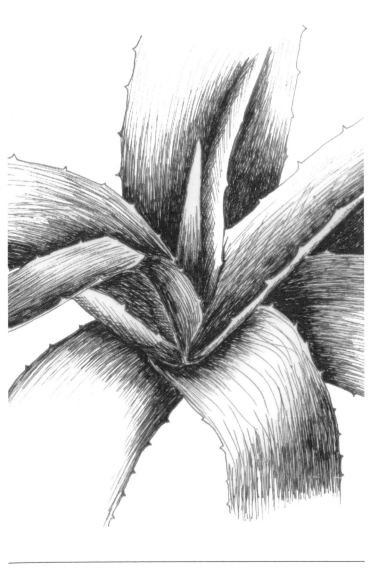

FLAX SEED HAIR GEL

This natural hair gel will not flake or make the hair stiff.
It is safe to use every day.

You will need: **Makes about 180 ml (6 fl oz)**

120 ml (4 fl oz) water
15 ml (1 tbsp) flax seeds
45 ml (3 tbsp) Aloe Vera gel
few drops fragrance oil of your choice

Method:

1. In a small saucepan, bring the water to the boil. Stir
in the flax seeds and reduce the heat. Simmer for about
10 minutes, stirring constantly until a gel-like lotion is
formed.
2. Remove from the heat and strain through a fine sieve
or cheesecloth into a bowl.
3. Add the Aloe Vera and fragrance oil and blend
thoroughly.
4. Pour into a cosmetic bottle and refrigerate for up to a
week.
5. Use as you would any other hair gel.

MOISTURISING SHAMPOO FOR DRY HAIR

You will need: **Makes 125 ml (about 4 fl oz)**

    60 ml (2 fl oz) mild liquid soap
    60 ml (2 fl oz) Aloe Vera gel
    5 ml (1 tsp) glycerine
    1.25 ml (¼ tsp) avocado oil

Method:

1. Mix all the ingredients together in a small bowl.
2. Pour into a pump-type cosmetic bottle.
3. Shake well before using. Apply to hair from root to tip and leave in for a few minutes.
4. Rinse well with cool water.

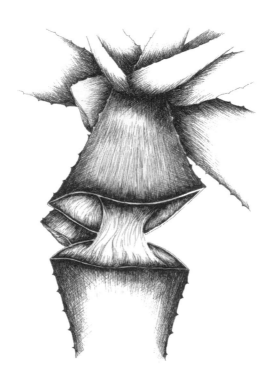

GRAPEFRUIT SHAMPOO BOOSTER FOR OILY HAIR

You will need: **Makes enough for two shampoos**

2.5 ml (½ tsp) Aloe Vera gel
15 ml (1 tbsp) grapefruit juice
60 ml (4 tbsp) mild shampoo

Method:

1. Mix the ingredients together in a small bowl and pour into a shampoo bottle.
2. Wash your hair using half of the mixture and rinse well.

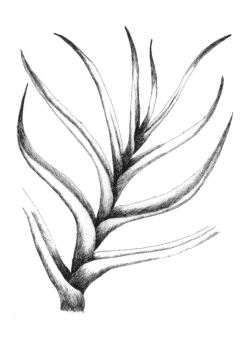

AFTER SUN RELIEF

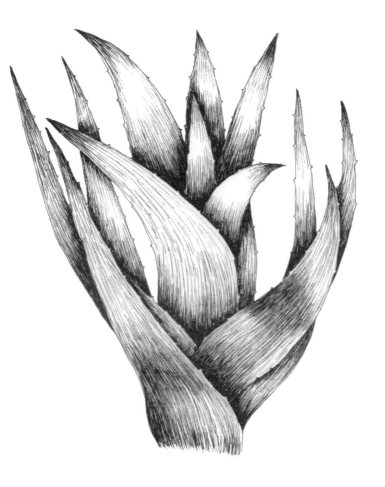

AFTERSUN RELIEF GEL NO.1

You will need: **Makes enough for one treatment**

3 drops lavender essential oil
brewed chamomile tea or green tea
30 ml (2 tbsp) Aloe Vera gel (or roughly the amount
extracted from one fresh leaf)

Method:

1. Mix essential oil, tea and Aloe Vera in a clean glass
bowl.
2. Apply with clean fingers directly onto sunburned or
mildly irritated skin. Use immediately. Do not store.

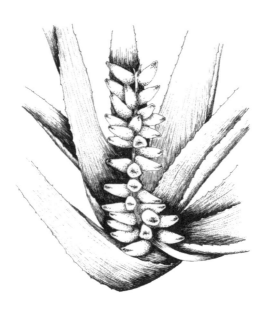

AFTERSUN RELIEF GEL NO. 2

You will need: **Makes 38 ml (about 1¼ fl oz)**

30 ml (2 tbsp) witch hazel
5 ml (1 tsp) glycerine
2.5 ml (½ tsp) kelp powder
2 drops chamomile essential oil
2 drops lavender essential oil

Method:

1. Blend the ingredients together and decant into a dark glass (recommended) or plastic dispenser bottle.
2. It is best stored in a cool place, where it will last approximately 3 months.
3. Shake well before use.

AFTERSUN RELIEF GEL NO. 3

You will need: **Makes about 300 ml (about 10 fl oz)**

1 roughly chopped cucumber
30 ml (2 tbsp) Aloe Vera gel (or roughly the amount
extracted from one fresh leaf)
60 ml (4 tbsp) glycerine
60 ml (4 tbsp) rosewater
2 drops rose essential oil

Method:

1. Place cucumber into a juicer or garlic press to extract
as much juice as possible.
2. Press through a sieve and reserve the liquid. Discard
the solids.
3. Mix the cucumber juice with the remaining
ingredients.
4. Store in the refrigerator for up to 3 days.

ALOE SUNBURN SPRAY

You will need: **Makes about 150 ml (5 fl oz)**

    15 drops lavender essential oil
    5 ml (1 tsp) vitamin E oil
    5 ml (1 tsp) vinegar
    120 ml (4 fl oz) Aloe Vera gel

Method:

1. Mix together all ingredients in a glass bowl.
2. Pour into a suitable cosmetic spray bottle.
3. Store in the refrigerator.

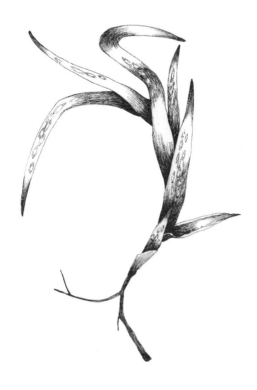

AFTERSUN SKIN GEL

You will need: **Makes 125 ml (about 4 fl oz)**

    100 ml (3½ fl oz) Aloe Vera gel
    20 ml (4 tsp) witch hazel
    5 ml (1 tsp) deodorised kelp powder
    5 drops chamomile essential oil
    5 drops lavender essential oil
    5 drops peppermint essential oil

Method:

1. Blend all ingredients together in a small bowl using an electric hand mixer or wire whisk.
2. Pour into glass roll-on bottles and keep in a cool, dark location out of direct sunlight.
3. Shake well before using.

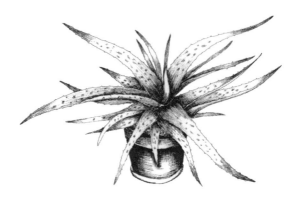

LIP GLOSS

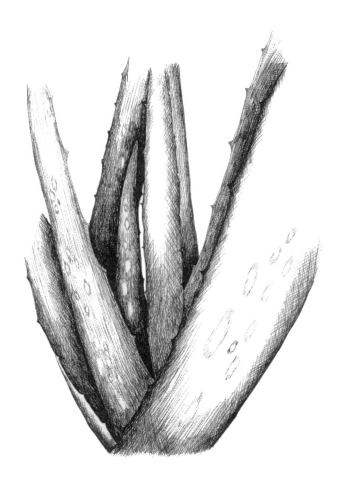

ALOE VERA LIP GLOSS

You will need: **Makes 12 ml (2½ tsp)**

    5 ml (1 tsp) Aloe Vera gel
    2.5 ml (½ tsp) virgin coconut oil
    5 ml (1 tsp) petroleum jelly (Vaseline) or
        non-petroleum jelly

Method:

1. Place ingredients in a small clean glass bowl and microwave for 1–2 minutes on high until melted. Stir to blend.
2. Pour into a small cosmetic container and cool.

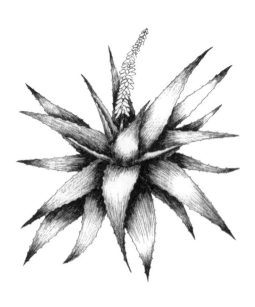

DELICIOUS TANGERINE LIP GLOSS

This make-it-yourself citrus lip gloss tastes lick-your-lips delicious, with both tangerine and lemon essential oils offering their benefits and flavours.

Tangerine essential oil is a bit of an aphrodisiac, so it is nice to wear out on a special date. The essential oils and honey combined make the gloss a tasty product that will keep your lips soft and moist for some time.

All the ingredients for this formula are easily found in health food stores or on the internet and the formula only takes about 10 minutes to make, so why not give it a try?

You will need: **Makes 65 ml (about 2½ fl oz)**

> 45 ml (3 tbsp) almond oil
> 15 g (½ oz) beeswax pellets
> 5 ml (1 tsp) Aloe Vera gel
> 5 ml (1 tsp) honey
> 2 x 400 IU vitamin E capsules
> 4 drops lemon essential oil
> 3 drops tangerine essential oil

Method:

1. Microwave the beeswax and sweet almond oil together in a glass bowl until melted.
2. Add the honey. Squeeze the vitamin E capsules into the bowl and mix briskly with a wire whisk.
3. Add the Aloe Vera gel and stir into the mixture.
4. Add the essential oils and stir in well.
5. Pour into a shallow cosmetic jar and apply as desired.

VANILLA LIP GLOSS

You will need: **Makes 45 ml (1½ fl oz)**

22 ml (1½ tbsp) petroleum jelly (Vaseline)
   or non-petroleum jelly
15 ml (1 tbsp) Aloe Vera gel
5 ml (1 tsp) almond oil
2.5 ml (½ tsp) vanilla essence (see below)

Method:

1. Combine ingredients in a glass bowl and microwave on low heat for 1 minute, stir and heat for another 20 seconds and stir again.
2. Scoop the mixture into shallow cosmetic pots and place in the refrigerator to harden slightly.

Note: You can vary the flavours of this lovely lip gloss by using different essences — try coffee or almond.

SKIN DISORDERS

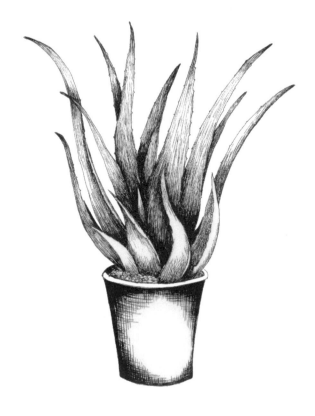

ACNE FACIAL MASK

You will need: **Makes enough for one treatment**

    7.5 ml (1½ tsp) cosmetic clay
    2.5 ml (½ tsp) marshmallow root powder
    2.5 ml (½ tsp) Aloe Vera gel
    1.25 ml (¼ tsp) witch hazel
    1 drop tea tree essential oil
    Distilled water

Method:

1. In a small bowl mix the cosmetic clay, marshmallow root, Aloe Vera, witch hazel and tea tree oil together.
2. Add water by the spoonful until it is the desired consistency.
3. To use, apply to face and leave on for 10 minutes or until the clay has dried.
4. Rinse off with warm water.

ALOE ACNE TREATMENT

Aloe Vera is a natural antibacterial and anti-inflammatory plant. Buy only pure Aloe Vera gel (or squeeze the gel from a fresh leaf) and apply it topically as needed. Aloe Vera helps to heal wounds of all kinds. If you have spots, gently cleanse your face with tea tree oil soap, pat dry, and apply Aloe Vera gel afterwards.

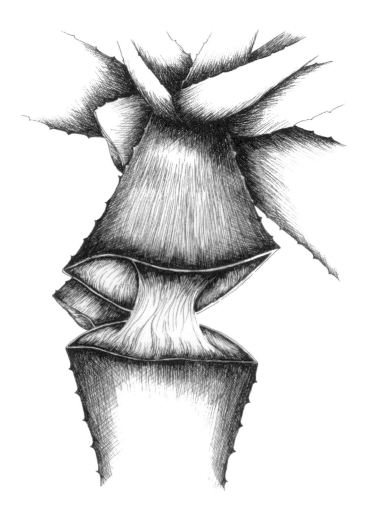

DRY SKIN TIRAMISU

You will need: **Makes enough for one treatment**

15 ml (1 tbsp) jojoba oil
15 ml (1 tbsp) sesame seed oil
Oil from 3 vitamin E capsules or 1.25 ml (¼ tsp) vitamin E
    base oil
10—15 ml (2—3 tsp) Aloe Vera gel

Method:

1. Mix the jojoba and sesame seed oil together in a small dish. Add the vitamin E oil and Aloe Vera and blend.
2. Apply to damp skin after you come out of the shower or bath to lock in moisture.

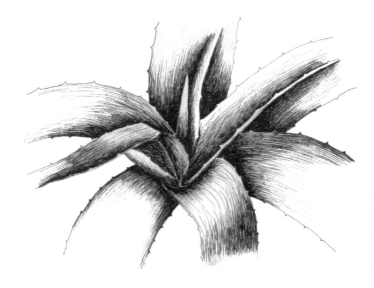

SKIN OINTMENT FOR SCARS

You will need: **Makes enough for one treatment**

7.5 ml (1½ tsp) Aloe Vera gel
10 ml (2 tsp) calendula cream or aqueous cream
1 vitamin E capsule

Method:

1. Mix the Aloe Vera with the calendula or aqueous cream in a small dish.
2. Break the vitamin E capsule into the bowl and mix well.
3. Apply to the wound. This works best when the scar is still healing.

OTHER ALOE APPLICATIONS

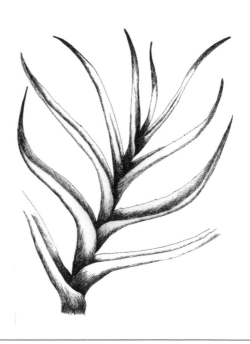

ALOE AFTERSHAVE GEL

This recipe will work well for both men and women. It is one of those simple recipes that will replace what you can buy in the shops. It soothes skin after you have finished shaving and it's alcohol-free, so it's great even for sensitive skin.

You will need: **Makes 160 ml (about 5¼ fl oz)**

120 ml (4 fl oz) Aloe Vera gel
25 ml (1½ tbsp) distilled or filtered water
15 ml (1 tbsp) witch hazel
10 drops essential oil or fragrance oil of your choice

Method:

1. Combine all ingredients well and pour into a lidded cosmetic container.
2. Use after every shave to soothe and revitalise your skin.

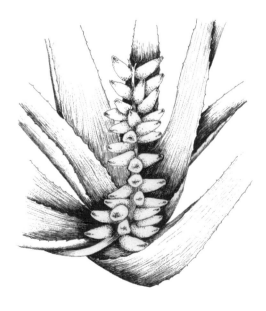

BUBBLEGUM ALOE HAND WIPE GEL

The kids will love to wipe their hands with this!

You will need: **Makes 180 ml (6 fl oz)**

120 ml (4 fl oz) Aloe Vera gel
60 ml (4 tbsp) surgical spirit
2.5 ml (½ tsp) bubblegum fragrance oil or other fragrance
oil of your choice

Method:

1. Mix all ingredients together in a small bowl.
2. Pour into a pump-style cosmetic bottle.
3. Take it along to picnics or other outdoor activities to clean your hands.
4. To use, dispense a small dollop onto the palm of your hand and rub hands together until the gel disappears. If necessary, wipe your hands with a tissue or paper towel.

TROPICAL DEODORANT LOTION

You will need: **Makes approximately 40 ml (1½ oz)**

12 ml (2½ tsp) Aloe Vera gel
10 ml (2 tsp) virgin coconut oil
10 ml (2 tsp) bicarbonate of soda
10 ml (2 tsp) arrowroot or cornflour
10 drops tea tree essential oil
10 drops lemon essential oil

Method:

1. Mix all ingredients together in a clean dish. The consistency will be runny.
2. Pour into a small clean cosmetic bottle and use a pea-sized amount per armpit.

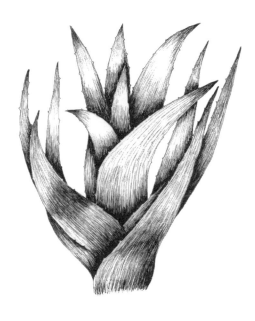

COCO DEODORANT CREAM

You will need: **Makes about 40 ml (1½ oz)**

10 ml (2 tsp) cocoa butter flakes
7.5 ml (1½ tsp) virgin coconut oil
2.5 ml (½ tsp) shea butter
10 ml (2 tsp) Aloe Vera gel
10 ml (2 tsp) cornflour
2.5 ml (½ tsp) bicarbonate of soda
10 drops lavender essential oil
4 drops tea tree essential oil

Method:

1. Mix the cocoa butter flakes with the coconut oil and shea butter in a small ramekin, then add the Aloe Vera gel and stir until well blended.
2. Add the cornflour and bicarbonate of soda and mix well. Add the essential oils.
3. Transfer to a small clean cosmetic jar and use as necessary.

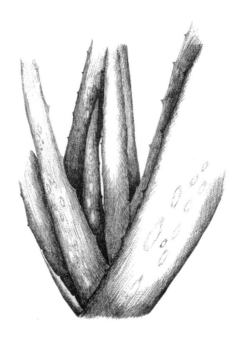

BABY AND HAND WIPES

Here are some ideas for homemade baby/hand wipes using paper towels or cloth nappies.

ALOE TEA TREE WIPES

You will need: **Makes 600 ml (1 pint)**

2 drops tea tree essential oil
90 ml (3 fl oz) liquid baby soap
60 ml (4 tbsp) Aloe Vera gel
450 ml (¾ pint) boiled water

ANTI-FUNGAL WIPES

(TO DISCOURAGE NAPPY RASH)

You will need: **Makes 375 ml (12½ fl oz)**

15 ml (1 tbsp) calendula oil
2 drops lavender essential oil or chamomile oil
2 drops tea tree essential oil or grapeseed extract
45 ml (3 tbsp) liquid baby soap
15 ml (1 tbsp) distilled vinegar (omit if baby has a raw nappy rash)
60 ml (4 tbsp) Aloe Vera gel
240 ml (8 fl oz) boiled water

Method:

1. Allow to cool and then mix water/ingredients together in a bowl.
2. Pour into a sterilised lidded bottle and store any extra solution in the fridge.

Most baby wipe solution recipes contain similar main ingredients, which are used for the same reason in each recipe. These are the common ingredients and why they are included:

- Oil: Helps the wipe glide across baby's skin and keeps skin soft.
- Soap: Cleanses by removing all traces of urine and faeces.
- Essential oils: added for antibacterial and/or aromatherapy purposes.
- Water: The main ingredient in each recipe, cleanses the nappy area and dilutes the other ingredients.

The type and amounts of oil, soap, essential oils and water that go into a recipe is what gives each wipe solution its own distinct 'personality'. Have fun trying different recipes until you find the ones that you like best.

HOW TO USE THESE SOLUTIONS

You may use either absorbent paper towels or cloth nappies or muslin squares cut to size.

When mixing solutions it works best to start with oil and end with water. The oil will coat your measuring tools so the soap slips right off. Be sure to add the water slowly or you'll end up with a ton of bubbles!

There are many different ways to store and apply baby wipe solutions; try a few of the following ideas to find the one that works best for your family. You may discover that one system works well at home and another works away from home. Most of the time it is easiest to gently mix the cloth wipe solution in a bottle with a cover and then pour it into a storage container.

- Use a spray bottle to moisten the baby wipes.
- Use a sports drink bottle with a pull-up spout to dribble solution onto the wipes.
- Warm the solution and put into an insulated container to provide warm wipes for your baby.

- Place cloth wipes in a commercial baby wipes container and pour wipes solution over wipes.
- Place the solution into a commercial baby wipes container and dip the wipes into the solution.

Note: Don't store solution or wet wipes for a long time because they can become musty and the wet wipes may even get mildewy. Check your solution and wet wipes daily, and mix smaller batches of solution frequently instead of large batches less often to avoid mustiness.

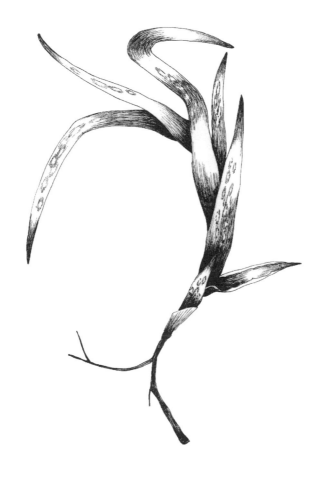

ALOE BROWN SUGAR BODY SCRUB

You will need: **Makes enough for one treatment**

   30 ml (2 tbsp) porridge oats
   30 ml (2 tbsp) brown sugar
   30 ml (2 tbsp) Aloe Vera gel
   15 ml (1 tbsp) runny honey
   5 ml (1 tsp) lemon juice
   5 ml (1 tsp) almond oil

Method:

1. Process the porridge oats and brown sugar to a powder in a blender or spice grinder.
2. Combine with the Aloe Vera, honey, lemon juice and almond oil in a small bowl.
3. Use as a body scrub prior to bathing.

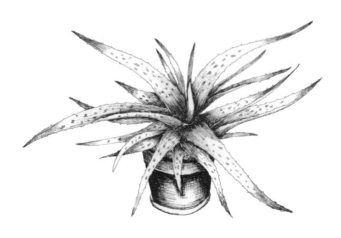

BUGS BEGONE! SPRAY

Catnip is a great treat for cats, but a big turn-off for mosquitoes.

You will need: **Makes 60 ml (2 fl oz)**

10 ml (2 tsp) Aloe Vera gel
30 ml (2 tbsp) witch hazel
10 ml (2 tsp) vodka
10 ml (2 tsp) distilled or filtered water
15 drops catnip essential oil
5 drops geranium essential oil (optional)

Method:

1. Blend all ingredients together in a small dish.
2. Pour into a spray cosmetic bottle.
3. Shake well before use.
4. Store in a cool, dark location.

BUGS BEGONE! SKIN GEL

You will need: **Makes 125 ml (about 4 fl oz)**

25 ml (5 tsp) Aloe Vera gel
75 ml (2½ fl oz) witch hazel
25 ml (5 tsp) distilled or filtered water
5 ml (1 tsp) deodorised kelp powder
20 drops catnip essential oil
5 drops geranium essential oil

Method:

1. Whisk all ingredients together in a glass bowl until kelp powder is dissolved.
2. Pour into cosmetic bottles or roll-on cosmetic bottles for easy dispensing.
3. Store in a cool, dark location.

CUCUMBER EYE GEL

You will need: **Makes about 60 ml (2 fl oz)**

¼ large cucumber, roughly chopped
30 ml (2 tbsp) Aloe Vera gel

Method:

1. Purée the cucumber in a blender or spice grinder.
2. Strain into a glass bowl and add a little of the cucumber pulp.
3. Mix in the Aloe Vera and stir to combine.
4. Pour the mixture into a clean cosmetic container.
5. Use after cleansing your face, applying with a cotton pad or ball to the area underneath your eyes. Avoid getting it into your eyes.
6. Store any unused portion of the gel in the refrigerator, but only keep for a few days because of the fresh cucumber.

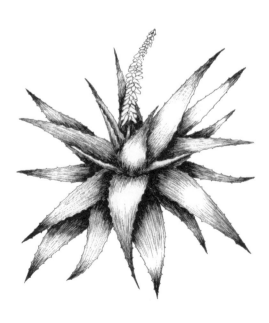

FAIRY DUST GLITTER GEL

Kids really love this trendy gel! It's also fun for adults and it's so easy to make.

You will need:

60 ml (4 tbsp) Aloe Vera gel
5 ml (1 tsp) glycerine
1.25 ml (¼ tsp) fine polyester glitter (any colour)*
5 drops fragrance oil (optional)
1 drop liquid food colouring (optional)

Method:

1. Mix the Aloe Vera gel and glycerine together in a small bowl. Stir in the polyester glitter and optional fragrance oil and food colouring. Scoop into a lidded cosmetic jar. That's it. It is now ready for use whenever you want to sparkle.

*Polyester glitter is available on the internet and from some speciality craft shops.

GRAPEFRUIT MASSAGE TONING OIL

When you are losing weight and want to tone your skin, try this. Grapefruit is said to stimulate detoxification.

You will need: **Makes 125 ml (about 4 fl oz)**

   15 drops grapefruit essential oil
   5 ml (1 tsp) olive oil
   120 ml (4 fl oz) Aloe Vera gel

Method:

1. Mix the ingredients together in a glass bowl.
2. Scoop into a suitable cosmetic container. Store in the refrigerator.
3. To use, massage into areas of the body that need toning.

GREEN APPLE SHOWER GEL

You will need: **Makes about 300 ml (10 fl oz)**

180 ml (6 fl oz) distilled water
120 ml (4 fl oz) unscented shampoo
30 ml (2 tbsp) Aloe Vera gel
5 ml (1 tsp) fine sea salt
15 drops green apple fragrance oil
1 drop green food colouring (optional)

Method:

1. Microwave the water in a glass bowl for about
1 minute until it is warm.
2. Add the shampoo to the bowl and stir until it is well
blended.
3. Add the Aloe Vera gel, salt, fragrance oil and green
colouring, if using. Stir until thick and well blended.
4. Pour into a clean plastic squeeze bottle and close
tightly.

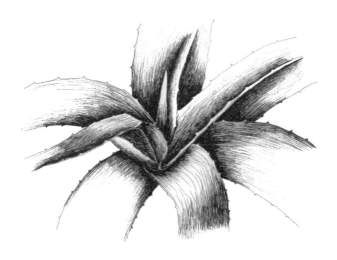

TRAVELLER'S FRIEND

When you are travelling, wrap a leaf of Aloe Vera in clingfilm and keep in your toilet kit.Better still, make up this potion:

You will need:

> 60 ml (2 fl oz) Aloe Vera gel, approximate amount of gel
>> extracted from two Aloe Vera leaves
> 6 vitamin E capsules

Method:

1. Mix the Aloe Vera gel with the contents of the vitamin E capsules in a small dish.
2. Transfer to a small dark cosmetic container and keep in your handbag or briefcase, or better still, in the refrigerator, until needed.

Culinary
Recipes

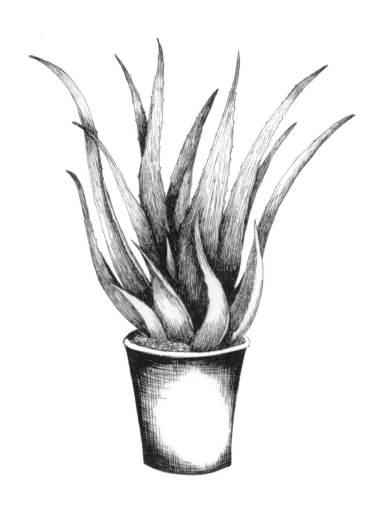

Aloe Vera gel is a very popular culinary ingredient in China, Japan and other Asian countries, and many products are already prepared, such as tinned Aloe Vera and Aloe Vera with yogurt, which is quite a popular dessert in some quarters. As far as I know, only the smoothies and some of the drinks appeal to Western tastes, but I am including a few recipes mainly for their ethnic flavour. Who knows? You may decide you like them.

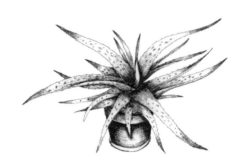

RECIPES

APPLE ALOE CUCUMBER DRINK

A fabulously healthy juice drink from down under. Make this when you are feeling a bit low.

You will need: **Serves 4**

   1 whole cucumber, cut into chunks
   2 tart apples, such as granny smith, peeled and cored
   Juice of 1 lemon
   60 ml (4 tbsp) aloe vera gel

Method:

1. Place the cucumber and apples in a blender and process until smooth.
2. Add the lemon juice and Aloe Vera gel.
3. Refrigerate or pour into tall glasses and add ice cubes.

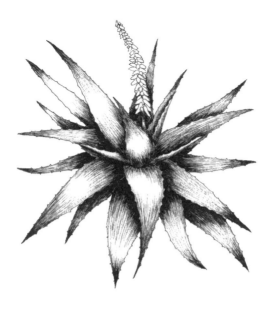

AWESOME FRUIT SMOOTHIE

This is a great breakfast smoothie, rich in vitamins, antioxidants, fibre, omega-3, monounsaturated fats, soy protein and much more. A wonderful way to start your day!

You will need: Serves 6

1 banana
½ apple
1 kiwi fruit
55 g (2 oz) frozen mixed berries
240 ml (8 fl oz) freshly squeezed orange juice
120 ml (4 fl oz) soy, oat or rice milk
115 g (4 oz) plain yogurt
100 g (3½ oz) silken tofu
45 ml (3 tbsp) natural unsalted peanut butter
30 ml (2 tbsp) Aloe Vera juice
30 ml (2 tbsp) flaxseed oil
5 ml (1 tsp) wheatgrass powder (optional)

Method:

1. In a blender combine the banana, apple, kiwi, berries and orange juice and blend until smooth.
2. Add the soy milk, yogurt, tofu, peanut butter, Aloe Vera juice, flaxseed oil and wheatgrass powder, if using, and blend again until everything is well mixed.
3. Pour into tall glasses and enjoy.

CHICKEN SOUP WITH ALOE

You will need: **Serves 4**

3 plump Aloe Vera leaves
700 g (1½ lb) chicken thighs, chopped into chunks
15 white peppercorns, crushed
3 dates, stones removed
1.2 litres (2 pints) water
Salt to taste

Method:

1. Wash the Aloe Vera leaves. Peel off the skin and cut the gel into thick slices. Set aside.
2. Poach the chicken, peppercorns and dates in the measured water for 1–1½ hours, until the chicken is very tender.
3. Add the Aloe Vera slices and continue to cook for an additional 20 minutes.
4. Season to taste, then serve hot.

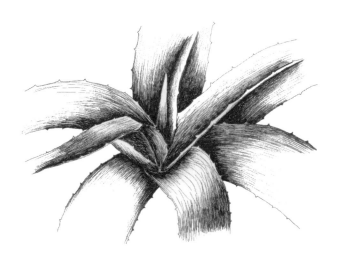

CHILLI FOR A CROWD

You will need: **Makes about 3.2 litres (5¼ pints)**

450 g (1 lb) freshly minced lean beef, turkey or chicken
3 x 400 g (14 oz) tins tomatoes
400 g (14 oz) tin red kidney beans
400 g (14 oz) tin black beans
400 g (14 oz) tin haricot or flageolet beans
400 g (14 oz) tin sweetcorn
3 bay leaves
240 ml (8 fl oz) lemon juice
45 ml (3 tbsp) Worcestershire sauce
180 ml (6 fl oz) Aloe Vera juice
10–12 chilli peppers (or to taste)
60 ml (4 tbsp) cayenne pepper (or to taste)
45 ml (3 tbsp) coarsely ground black pepper
Cooked rice, to serve
Crusty bread, to serve

Method:

1. In a small frying pan, brown the beef, turkey or chicken and drain the fat.
2. Place into a large stewpot and add the tomatoes, beans and sweetcorn.
3. Add the bay leaves, lemon juice, Worcestershire sauce and Aloe Vera juice. Mix to blend.
4. Add the chilli peppers, cayenne pepper and black pepper. Be careful. You can always add more later.
5. Bring to the boil over a medium heat. Cover and reduce the heat to a simmer and cook for about 2 hours.
6. Check the seasoning, remove from the heat and serve over rice with crusty bread.
7. Leftovers can be cooled, refrigerated and reheated. But be sure you heat it all the way through.

CHINESE CONGEE WITH ALOE VERA

You will need:　　　　　　　　　　　**Serves 6 to 8**

180 g (6 oz) long grain rice
2.4 litres (3½ pints) water
5 ml (1 tsp) salt
115 g (4 oz) cooked pork or chicken, shredded
55 g (2 oz) cooked mushrooms, diced
2 spring onions, white and green parts, sliced
115 g (4 oz) Aloe Vera gel from the leaf or tinned, diced

Method:

1. In a large saucepan, bring the rice, water and salt to the boil.
2. Reduce the heat to low, cover the pan and cook on a low heat, stirring occasionally until the rice has the thick, creamy texture of porridge, about 1 hour.
3. Remove from the heat and stir in the pork or chicken, mushrooms, spring onions and Aloe Vera.
4. Place the pan back on a low heat until just heated through.
5. Serve immediately.

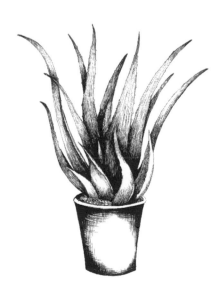

ENDERONG DELIGHT

You will need: **Serves 8**

    1 stalk (20 cm/8 inches) lemongrass, cut into small pieces
    Juice of 4 limes
    30 ml (2 tbsp) water for the syrup
    200 g (7 oz) sugar
    4 passion fruits
    1 small slice of fresh ginger
    1 piece of Aloe Vera (about 4 cm/1½ inches long)
    1.2 litres (1¾ pints) water

Method:

1. Put the lemongrass, lime juice, and water for the syrup in a saucepan over a low heat. Stir the mixture gently with a wooden spoon until the sugar is melted. Let it simmer for 5 more minutes. Remove from the heat and let it stand covered for 10 minutes.
2. Cut open the passion fruits and scoop out the flesh. Skin the Aloe Vera, put them both into a blender and add 200 ml (7 fl oz) water. Blend the mixture on high speed, then strain it or not as you like (some prefer to drink it with the residue of the passion fruit seeds which are high in fibre) and pour into a jug.
3. Strain the reserved lemongrass syrup and pour it into the passion fruit juice, add the remaining water and serve with crushed ice.

CUCUMBER AND GINGER FIZZ

You will need: **Makes 6—8 servings**

170 g (6 oz) granulated sugar
180 ml (6 fl oz) water
225 g (8 oz) fresh ginger, cut into 5 cm (2 inch) chunks
60 ml (4 tbsp) fresh basil, chopped
2 large cucumbers
540 ml (18 fl oz) sparkling water
60 ml (4 tbsp) Aloe Vera juice
Basil leaves to garnish

Method:

1. First make the ginger and basil syrup. In a saucepan over a medium heat, bring the sugar and water to a boil.
2. Meanwhile, place the ginger and basil in a blender and process.
3. Add the ginger-basil mixture to the sugar syrup and simmer for 30 minutes. Remove from the heat, strain and cool.
4. Chop 1½ cucumbers and put into the blender with a dash of sparkling water and process. Mix with the remainder of the sparkling water and Aloe Vera juice.
5. To serve, fill tall glasses with ice. Add 60—90 ml (2—3 fl oz) ginger-basil syrup to each glass and top up with the sparkling water mixture. Garnish with a round of cucumber and basil leaves.

HONEY LEMON ALOE VERA FRUIT SALAD

You will need: **Serves at least 8—10**

1 stalk of fresh organic Aloe Vera (approx. 675 g/1½ lb)
150 ml (5 fl oz) pure organic honey
½ unwaxed lemon, cut into wedges
Peaches, strawberries or oranges to serve

Method:

1. Wash the Aloe Vera, remove the skin and cut the flesh into small cubes. Tip into a bowl.
2. Add the honey and lemon wedges and mix well.
4. Refrigerate the mixture for at least one hour for the gel to settle and become watery.
5. Just before serving, add other fruits such as peaches, strawberries or oranges.

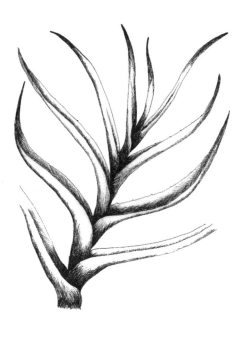

PEACH ALOE SMOOTHIE

You will need: **Serves 2**

    3 fresh peaches, stoned and sliced (leave skin on)
    15 ml (1 tbsp) ground cinnamon
    2.5 ml (½ tsp) ginseng extract
    2.5 ml (½ tsp) Aloe Vera gel
    2 cloves (optional)

Method:

1. Mix ingredients in a blender, whizzing until smooth, taking care to stop the machine at intervals and scrape down the sides to ensure proper blending.
2. Chill in the refrigerator until ready to serve.
3. Pour into tall glasses and add ice cubes if desired.

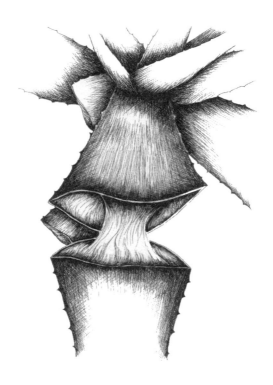

WONTON SOUP

You will need: **Serves 4**

    1 large slice Aloe Vera gel, skin removed and cut into
       small cubes
    250 g (9 oz) minced pork or minced raw prawns
    18—24 wonton wrappers
    1.2 litres (2 pints) vegetable stock
    Rice noodles (optional)

Method:

1. In a bowl, mix the Aloe Vera with the minced pork or
prawns.
2. Lay the wonton wrappers out on a work surface and
place a spoonful of the pork-Aloe filling in the centre of
each wrapper. Twist each side of the wrapper to seal.
3. Bring a large pan of water to the boil and boil the
wontons for 5—8 minutes until the filling is cooked.
Remove the wontons with a slotted spoon.
4. In another large saucepan, heat the vegetable stock
until it comes to the boil. Add the rice noodles, if using,
and boil for 3 minutes. Add the wontons. When the
wontons float to the top of the pan, the soup is ready.
5. Serve immediately.

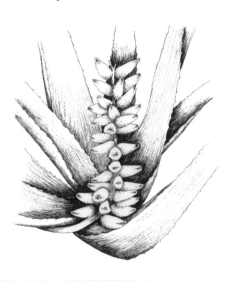

Glossary

Acemannan
A complex carbo-hydrate considered to be one of the major ingredients in Aloe Vera.

Aloe Barbadensis Aloe barbadensis is the main species of what we call Aloe Vera (true aloe).

Aloin A bitter, yellow crystalline compound obtained from Aloe Vera and used as a laxative.

Alopecia Loss of hair, baldness.

Aloe Vera Gel Parenchymal tissue obtained from the peeled leaves of Aloe Barbadensis.

Aloe Vera Latex The bitter, yellow liquid contained in the rind of Aloe Barbadensis, the principal constituent of which is aloin.

Amino acids The building blocks of proteins.

Anthraquinone Occurs naturally in Aloe Vera and other plants. Helps provide colour of plant and is one of the key ingredients when Aloe Vera is used as a laxative.

Antifungal Destroying or inhibiting the growth of funguses.

Anti-inflammatory Preventing or reducing inflammation.

Antioxidant In the case of Aloe Vera, thought to protect body cells from the damaging effects of oxidation.

Antiseptic Capable of preventing infection by inhibiting the growth of disease-causing micro-organisms.

Antiviral Destroying or inhibiting the growth of reproduction of viruses.

Ayurvedic medicine The ancient Hindu science of health and medicine.

AZT A major drug used in the treatment of HIV (AIDS).

Beta Sitosterol A chemical structure that mimics cholesterol and is used to reduce LDL (bad fat) in the bloodstream.

Body Mass Index (BMI) A measure of the percentage of fat and muscle in the body, used as an indicator of ideal weight.

Cholesterol Divided into HDL (good fat) and LDL (bad fat) to indicate heart health.

Collagen The constituent of skin that makes skin look plumper and less wrinkled.

CoQ10 A naturally occurring nutrient in the body with antioxidant properties.

Cortisone A steroid used in the treatment of arthritis.

Detoxification The process of cleansing the body of toxins (poisons).

Enzyme Any of numerous proteins functioning as catalysts enabling chain reactions.

Epithelium Membrane Tissue forming the covering of most internal and external surfaces of the body and its organs.

Herpes Zoster (Shingles) A very painful viral skin infection usually contracted by those who have had chickenpox.

Hyperlipidaemia An excess of fats or lipids in the blood.

Hypoglycaemia Low blood sugar.

Leukaemia A form of cancer attacking the bone marrow and blood cells.

Micronutrient A substance such as vitamin or mineral essential in minute amounts essential for the growth of organisms.

Monosaccharide Any of several carbo-hydrates unable to be broken down by hydrolysis, also called simple sugar.

Mucilage The gel sourced from the Aloe Vera plant.

Nucleoprotein Any of a group of complexes of protein and nucleic acid found in the cytoplasm of all living cells and in viruses.

Parenchyma The most common plant tissue — in this instance, the gel of Aloe Vera.

Pericyclic tubule Located between the endodermis (innermost layer of the plant) and the phloem.

Peripheral Neuropathy Disorder of the nervous system causing tingling in the hands and feet.

Phloem The living tissue that carries organic nutrients, particularly sucrose, a sugar, to all parts of the plant where needed.

Polypeptide A single linear chain of two or more amino acids.

Polysaccharide The form in which most natural carbohydrates occur.

Psyllium The seed husks are mainly used to relieve constipation, IBS, diverticular disease and diarrhoea.

Pulmonary Carcinogenesis The process which leads to the development of lung cancer.

Retrovirus Any of a group of viruses, many of which produce tumours, including the virus that causes AIDS.

Salicylic acid A crystalline acid used in the production of aspirin. Also used in external treatment of eczema.

Sarcoma A type of skin cancer.

Seborrhoea Disease of sebaceous glands caused by the overproduction of sebum.

Sludge blood A cluster of blood cells sticking together which impedes circulation.

SPF (Sun protection factor) The degree to which a sunscreen protects the skin from ultraviolet rays. Usually expressed numerically.

Statin Any of a class of lipid-lowering drugs to reduce cholesterol.

Taxonomy Classification of organisms.

Triglycerides are the chemical form in which most fat exists in food as well as in the body. They're also present in blood plasma and, in association with cholesterol, form the plasma lipids. When elevated, they are a factor, with cholesterol, in heart disease.

Xylem Woody tissue of vascular plants.

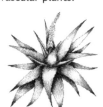